Medical Writing:

A Brief Guide for Beginners

Edited By:

Carol EH Scott-Conner MD PhD

To my husband, Harry F Conner MD MPH, for his unwavering love and support; and to my residents and colleagues, who continue to inspire and teach me.

Chapter authors:

Wei Chen MD
Plastic and Reconstructive Surgery
University of Iowa Carver College of Medicine

Kent Choi MD
Acute Care Surgery
University of Iowa Carver College of Medicine

Alice M Fagin MD
Arkansas Children's Hospital

Neelima Katragunta MD
Vascular Surgery
University of Iowa Carver College of Medicine

Scott Sherman MD
Department of Surgery
University of Iowa Carver College of Medicine

Manuscript Reviewers:

Alan Reed MD MBA
Transplantation and Hepatobiliary Surgery
University of Iowa Carver College of Medicine

Sonia Sugg MD
Surgical Oncology and Endocrine Surgery
University of Iowa Carver College of Medicine

Table of Contents

Introduction

This book is intended for health care professionals who are preparing to write their first paper for submission to a medical journal. Like many of the things that we do in medicine, writing is something you learn. Even if you were an English major in college, there are specific tricks and nuances to medical writing that can make or break your first attempts to become published.

The book provides a practical, systematic approach that has served me well. It reflects my own experience as an author, as well as a member of numerous editorial boards and editor-in-chief of a surgical journal (*"Surgical Laparoscopy, Endoscopy, and Percutaneous Techniques"*) and a medical literary journal (*"The Examined Life Journal"*).

I have taught this approach to countless medical students, residents, and junior faculty members over the past decades. It contains information that I wish I had known when I first started out. Many of these tips and hints were passed along to me by more experienced authors.

There are many excellent comprehensive texts that include information about experimental design, grant writing, data analysis, and presentation. Some of my favorites are listed in Chapter 15, Additional Recommended Resources. This book is intended to answer some practical questions that may seem too obvious to ask, and that are largely too simple to be included in those books. These are the questions that people knock on my door to ask.

In this book, I assume that you have clinical material or data that is ready to write up for publication. Perhaps your mentor has told you, "Go write it up." You don't even know where to start. Or, perhaps, you have been invited to write a review article with your mentor, and your mentor expects you to write the first draft. Again, you find yourself at a starting point. My goal is to help you put together a manuscript that presents your material fairly, honestly, and clearly. I also include pointers on how to select a journal, and what to do if your manuscript is rejected.

Separate volumes in my series will deal with writing and editing medical books (or book-length electronic resources), and with creative writing for medical professionals.

Think of this book as the friendly senior colleague down the hall, the one who answers those questions you might be embarrassed to ask your primary mentor or chair.

I wish you well in your career, and hope that this brief guide will help you get started. This print volume was produced for those who do not wish to use an e-book. In place of the live hyperlinks in the e-book, URL's have been detailed in the text wherever an electronic resource is cited. All URL's are correct as of October 2015. If you find one that has changed, or if you have questions that I did not address in this book, please contact me. Together we can make this book even better.

Carol EH Scott-Conner MD PhD
Carol-scott-conner@uiowa.edu
Emeritus Professor of Surgery
University of Iowa Carver College of Medicine

Chapter 1. When to Write

This chapter is about time - the phases of an academic career, and how writing contributes to academic development. When you write, you contribute to the vast archive of medical knowledge. When you are put up for promotion, the number and quality of your publications contribute to the weight of your CV. Sometimes it seems like publication comes easily to senior faculty, particularly those with well-funded laboratories and armies of graduate students or trainees. The important thing to realize is that they all started somewhere.

The first half of this chapter deals with academic career development. It sets the context for the material which is to follow. If you are a resident who is not planning an academic career, the first half of this chapter may seem irrelevant. Scan through it rapidly anyhow, as it may give you some insight into the environment in which you are seeking publication. If you aspire to, or are beginning, an academic career, I encourage you to read this section carefully.

The second part of this chapter is about the mechanics of finding the time to write and developing an organizational style that facilitates, rather than hinders, your efforts to write. This is a key issue for all writers.

Writing and the Phases of an Academic Career

Writing is a part of academic life, and the publishing venue that is chosen appears to parallel the development of a scholarly career. Many trainees and junior faculty begin with case reports and original research articles in their early years, and move naturally on to invited contributions such as book chapters later. Finally, perhaps, as senior faculty members, they may undertake to write or edit a book or monograph in which the best thinking in their field is synthesized and rendered accessible.

Alternatively, you may be given the task of drafting a review article or book chapter early in your career, if your mentor offers it to you. Or, you may start right off writing research reports, particularly if you choose to spend a significant amount of time actually doing bench, clinical, or outcomes research or if you pursue graduate training in a related subject in addition to your professional degree.

Achieving visibility in academics. In order to advance in academics, you need to develop an area of expertise. Ideally, all of your publications should build into this area. Think of building a tower, where every brick contributes to the height of the final structure. This does not mean that you should turn down opportunities to write in related areas. Most young writers who ultimately become highly productive will take advantage of any chance to get involved in a project. However, as your career advances, the best way to attain national and even international visibility is to become known in a narrow area. If one follows the analogy of building a tower, one would generally build the base wider (early publications) than the top (final area of specialization).

Writing is just part of achieving visibility. Professional organizations provide the structure in which networking outside your own department can occur. They also provide a venue for presentation and publication. There are several kinds of organizations, and most academic faculty members belong to more than one.

Types of organizations. Let's take surgery as an example. Academic surgeons tend to belong to multiple organizations, and ultimately aspire to be active in a subset of these. How do you know which organizations to join? As with many aspects of academia, there is no substitute for personal mentorship. Here is some general information that may be of help. Links to the current websites for these organizations are given at the end of the chapter.

Most young surgeons begin by joining the American College of Surgeons, perhaps initially as candidate members and then as Fellows. This is an example of a comprehensive or general (in the sense of including multiple subspecialties), national (really, international), organization. Because it is so large, involvement in the ACS typically begins at the state level or through one of the committees, such as the Commission on Cancer. It may take an entire career to achieve higher levels of visibility in the ACS. Regional surgical societies, such as the Central Surgical Association, provide extremely high quality meetings that also span a wide range of surgical topics and yet, by their more limited size, may provide an opportunity for a young surgeon to get involved sooner. Most academic surgeons also belong to the regional society which represents their geographic location.

Then there are national associations devoted to academic surgery, such as the Association of Academic Surgeons (AAS) and the Society of University Surgeons (SUS). They also hold annual meetings, which tend to be research-intensive as opposed to the more clinically-oriented meetings of the comprehensive or general organizations. They also sponsor short courses in academic development and leadership. Most academic surgeons belong to one or both; usually attaining admission to the AAS first, and then to the more competitive SUS.

Finally, there are specialty-specific organizations such as the American Association for the Surgery of Trauma (AAST), the Society of Surgical Oncologists (SSO), and the American Society of Breast Surgeons (ASBrS). These provide continuing education and opportunities to present research to a specialized audience.

Achieving visibility within organizations. Visibility comes from being there, doing the work that needs to be done, and being useful. Come to the annual meeting and participate (by presenting or discussing papers). Volunteer to be on a committee or ask a friend to nominate you. Once on a committee, work hard and contribute to the effort.

This may seem daunting at first. Even the simple act of walking up to a microphone during the annual meeting to ask a question of the presenter can be intimidating. Make it easy for the moderator and the audience by giving your name and institution first, rather than assuming people do or do not know who you are. Be prepared. Look over the abstracts on the way to the meeting and prepare one or two questions to ask. Ask questions that will genuinely illuminate or clarify important points. As you listen and observe what others do, you will undoubtedly see both good examples and bad examples. Don't stand up and give your own paper. Be brief, to the point, and then go sit down.

Choose one or two organizations to concentrate upon. For various reasons, you may find yourself a member of more organizations than you planned on joining. This often happens when you have more than one mentor, and each is enthusiastically pushing you to join his or her favorite group. It is impossible to go to all the annual meetings, or to participate in a meaningful fashion. Identify the most important ones for your own career focus. If your focus is breast surgery and your work is primarily clinical, the American Society of Breast Surgeons is an ideal fit. If, on the other hand, you are running a National Cancer Institute-funded laboratory in breast cancer research, you may find the Society of Surgical Oncology is the best fit for you. Many people who are active clinically and in research belong to both. If in doubt, ask your mentor, or ask various experienced faculty members in your discipline.

Talk to people at the receptions and dinners. Go up to someone who gave a paper and congratulate them on their research. Follow up with an email or exchange business cards, if it appears that you may have interests in common.
If this seems daunting, cruise the poster sessions. The person assigned to stand by the poster is often the person who did the actual work; and frequently that is someone relatively junior and therefore highly approachable. As you will learn when you, in turn, stand beside your poster, that person is probably wondering if *anyone* is going to stop and show some interest.

Writing and organizational membership. The annual meetings of various organizations provide several types of opportunities to present and publish material. Virtually all solicit original research (basic science or clinical) by annual calls for abstracts. Of perhaps 100 abstracts received, only 20 may be selected for podium (oral) presentation, with a larger number – perhaps 40 or 50 or even more – selected for poster presentation. Some meetings encourage submission of a manuscript at the time of presentation, others do not. This is an excellent way to get visibility for your research. In addition (see the section on Deadlines, below), the deadline to complete the manuscript has a wonderful way of prodding one on to completion.

As you develop visibility, you may be invited to teach in a postgraduate course or to participate in a panel discussion. Preparing for this session may not directly lead to publication, but is an excellent stimulus to review the literature. Having reviewed the literature, why not write a review article? The topic is likely to be timely (or you would not have been asked to speak about it).

Promotion and tenure. There are multiple tracks in academics. The traditional "tenure track" is becoming rare as people acknowledge how difficult it is to maintain a busy clinical practice and fulfill all the requirements. Promotion on the tenure track requires a solid body of scholarly writing, usually requires extramurally funded research, clinical excellence, and evidence of teaching and administration/service. As of this writing, fewer and fewer entry-level faculty positions are available on the tenure track at most institutions.

Various non-tenure tracks, such as the clinical track or the clinician-educator track, have requirements that emphasize clinical excellence and regional and national visibility, some publication (this may be optional) and administrative or educational visibility. Extramurally-funded research is generally not required.

It is imperative that you become familiar with the requirements for promotion in your track at your institution. Speak with your Division Director and/or Department Chair, and, if possible, the Dean of Faculty. Remember that expectations may vary from department to department, and may (appropriately) vary depending upon the role you are assigned within your department. Thus, for example, if you are the third year medical student clerkship director, the expectation for administration of this program and excellence (as a role model) in teaching become foremost. If you are the director of the Breast Center, administration and clinical excellence become paramount.

When you are put up for promotion, you will need external letters of reference. Ideally, these are people who did not train you and have not worked with you, but rather know you through your work. With that in mind, it is easy to see the importance of achieving regional and national visibility within organizations.

When to Consider Writing

First of all, obviously you should only write when you have something to say. But don't carry that to the extreme by waiting until you are ready to say all there is to say about a topic. Creativity is a wellspring; do not be afraid of exhausting your material. Think of writing as a muscle – it becomes stronger with use. Consider publishing if you have:

- unique clinical material
- a new technique to report
- an unusual complication or conjunction of findings (for example, AIDS in the early days)

- results (positive or negative) from a hypothesis-driven research study
- a synthesis of findings (chapter, monograph, review article, textbook)
- researched and found nothing in recent literature (a rediscovery)
- material to communicate to the public (for example, to raise awareness of male breast cancer)

Become familiar with the literature in your specialty. This may seem obvious, but it will give you a sense of the sorts of paper that are published in the journals commonly read by physicians of your specialty. It will also give you a sense of what is or has been described recently. Consider writing about something weird if you have never seen it described, even if it seems mundane (for example, edema of breast associated with venous hypertension from an A-V fistula).

Write when you perceive a need. Arthur C Guyton wrote his highly successful "Textbook of Medical Physiology" because he perceived for a text written for medical students rather than for physiologists. Generations of physicians benefited.

Two of my own textbooks, "Operative Anatomy" and "The SAGES Manual: Fundamentals of Laparoscopy and GI Endoscopy" were similarly written out of sense of frustration and need. Both have gone into multiple editions over the decades.

The rhythm of the academic year. The distinct rhythm of the academic year extends to the abstract submission and meeting calendar. Submitting abstracts to meetings that require a completed manuscript is one way to get writing. If your abstract is accepted, you will have about six to nine months to complete the manuscript. Accumulate a database of abstract deadlines, notification times, and dates of meetings. Meetings tend to be held in the spring and fall, with abstract deadlines around six to nine months ahead of the meeting. Thus, an association that meets in March might require abstracts by the end of August. The abstracts are then read, rated, and ranked by the publications committee and the final selections (and notification) may be made in October. Chapter 14 has more details on how to create, maintain, and use a calendar of abstract deadlines and meetings.

Your abstract may well be rejected, especially in the beginning. You can only submit to one meeting at a time, so you need to have a fallback plan. If you submit an abstract for a spring meeting, the logical fallback plan is to submit to the next appropriate abstract deadline (typically a winter or spring deadline for a meeting in the autumn). Do NOT submit the same material to two meetings at the same time. It is naïve to think you will not be found out, and it is easy to get a bad reputation in the relatively small world of academics.

Some meetings require a manuscript at the time of the meeting. This is great, because you now have a deadline to produce a full manuscript and some assurance that your paper will be seriously considered for publication. If the organization requires or encourages submission of a manuscript at the time of presentation, do so. The publications committee will review these manuscripts and then send them along to the journal for further editorial review. The process is discussed in more detail in Chapter 12. For now, the important point is that the odds of acceptance are much higher than if you simply sent the manuscript to the same journal without going through the meeting. This is because the organization will have an arrangement with that particular journal to devote a specific number of pages to papers from the annual meeting. There is no guarantee of acceptance, but acceptance of your abstract indicates a degree of interest and you are part of a much smaller pool competing for a limited number of pages in the journal. A handful of meetings guarantee publication, but this is exceedingly rare.

Even if no manuscript is solicited by the organization, go ahead and complete yours while the material is fresh in your mind. The material must not be published before you present it at the meeting, so be careful about submitting it to a journal.

Of course, once you have presented material at one meeting, you cannot submit it to another. The exception to this rule is when you are asked to give an invited address or a state of the art lecture, participate in a panel, or in some way present the body of knowledge in an area.

Finding Time to Write

Some people feel that they need to devote a specific block of time to writing. They will dedicate a specific time of day, or a part of a day of the week. This allows uninterrupted work, but presents a potential problem if you are unable to keep the "date with yourself" because of the press of clinical, administrative, or personal responsibilities. The pitfall here is that you just never get around to writing, because you don't have any "writing time."

I advocate instead that you learn how to use bits and pieces of time. Stitch these together to create blocks of time. Make your writing portable and you are all set to write during otherwise wasted time. In addition, by writing in short bursts, you may be less likely to run out of steam. A good general rule is to stop writing when it is still going well, rather than writing to exhaustion. If you stop while it is still going well and jot down a couple of notes on where you are going next, you are likely to find yourself eager to return to the job. You may also find that you are mulling over your writing project during odd moments during the day – the daily commute, for example – and solving problems that may have seemed daunting before.

Consider using early morning time on weekends or when you and your family are on vacation. Get up early and put in an hour or so writing. Or write when the rest of the family is off doing something you don't care to participate in. Find a nearby public library and sit down at a desk. You will be writing at a time when you are refreshed and much less distracted than when you are at work. Resist the temptation to say, "But that's *my* time!" It *is* your time, but this is a great way to use it.

Making your writing portable. To effectively use spare time, make your writing materials portable, and take them with you wherever you go. This is easy in the current era of tablet computers, but even lacking that, you can simply use index cards for your references and develop a file with the latest version of your manuscript, some notes, and a pad of paper or a spiral bound notebook. This allows you to use unexpected blocks of "down time" productively. Immediately back up anything your produce during your spare bits of time by saving it to "the cloud" or e-mailing it to yourself.

Maintain one "working copy." Although it is possible to merge changes from several versions of a document, you will probably find it simpler to just maintain one working copy. When you finish a writing session, save this copy (and back it up) and e-mail it to yourself. By e-mailing it yourself, it is available wherever you are.

Where to write. With portability, you will develop the ability to write anywhere. You may jot a few notes during an otherwise boring meeting, in the OR lounge while you are waiting for a case to start, or during unexpected gaps in clinic. You can write while sitting with your team in angiography as your trauma patient undergoes embolization.

If, on the other hand, you need to be in a specific place, you are back to the question of getting blocks of time in that place. If your special place is your desk at home, you need free time at home to sit at that desk and work. One strategy, if you are someone who really needs a definite time and a place, is to schedule some time to go to the medical library and sit and work. Plan when the work will be done and arrange the time and place accordingly.

In reality, most successful writers do both. They work on a project whenever they have a bit of free time, and they schedule and use blocks of time for concentrated work. Some phases of a writing project can be done piecemeal, a bit at a time, and some need thoughtful attention over an hour or more to achieve clarity.

When NOT to Write

Don't write just to get more papers out there. Remember the first cardinal rule – write when you have something to say.

The junior faculty member who is struggling to establish a research career should not take on too many invited contributions such as book chapters. In many universities, these are not counted toward promotion and tenure decisions. A well-done book chapter requires an inordinate amount of time, and is highly satisfying, but may not be the best use of your time. This is discussed more in the following chapter.

Chapter 2. Forms of Medical Writing

This chapter will introduce you to the various forms of medical writing, with particular focus on the difference between writing book chapters and other invited contributions versus journal articles. It also briefly deals with writing for a lay audience, and publishing on a website.

Book Chapters

The invitation to write a book chapter may fall to you relatively early in your career if, for example, a senior colleague has accepted an assignment and generously offers to include you in the project (or, more cynically, decides you are a cheap source of skilled labor). Usually this means that you will do the literature search and draft the chapter, with more or less guidance and approval from your senior author, and that both your names will appear on the final project. This can be a great way to get some personal mentoring from a more experienced author as well as a publication for your CV.

Before you automatically say, "I'd be delighted!" stop and think carefully. The primary question is: will this interfere with other, more critical commitments? In other words: are there better uses for your time? The following questions may help you decide.

Does the topic match your area of interest and expertise? As a junior faculty member, you may be invited to coauthor a chapter in your mentor's area of expertise. That area may or may not exactly match your own interests. The closer the match, the more easily you will be able to accomplish the task. On the other hand, taking on an assignment only peripherally related to your area of current specialization may open a whole new world of scholarship to you. Note that I said "area of current specialization." In fact, if you examine the CV's of prominent senior academics, it is not unusual to find that at various points in each career one topic or another may come into prominence, be explored in a series of publications, and then give way to the next.

Why say YES? Book chapters are by invitation only – thus, there is a certain prestige and automatic visibility, particularly if the chapter is part of a major textbook. It is an honor to be asked. Plus, maybe, your mentor asked you to do it.

Why say NO? You will need to allow several months (at least three) to properly research and write your chapter. More typically, it is a six month project. You will need to work to specifications (length, style, content) and to deadline. Take the specifications and the deadline seriously and honor them. Delay of a month or so in delivering the manuscript is usually acceptable (some would argue, even expected) but a greater delay risks delaying publication or even being excluded from the finished project. If you agree to do a chapter and then find that you cannot deliver on time, communicate this with the editor. Often the editor will be accommodating.

Here are two other factors to consider:

- Book chapters are not currently accessed by PubMed, hence any data that you include in a chapter is not accessible, but is considered "published." Do not put primary (original, unpublished) data in a chapter.
- Many institutions do not count book chapters (or even books) as original scholarship in promotion and tenure decisions. A chapter may help a faculty member on the clinical track, but not necessarily help another faculty member on the tenure track. Know what is expected of you on your academic career path and work accordingly!

Thus book chapters take a lot of time and may not be worth it for junior faculty. Only you can decide if the time is right for you to accept an invitation to contribute. If you decide to participate, honor your commitment. If you earn a reputation for delivering high quality material on time, you will be asked to contribute again. The contrary is also quite true. Every book editor has had the experience of having a chapter author confess, at the very last minute, that the chapter never got written.

How to write a book chapter. First, clearly establish the timeline and terms. Generally an author is allowed 6 months to complete a chapter and may enlist one or two coauthors. There is rarely any financial payment. Authors are generally given one or more complimentary copies of the finished book and may be allowed to buy additional copies (or other books published by the same firm) at the discount.

If you are working with a senior coauthor, make sure you understand how the work will be divided up, whose name will go first, and how you will collaborate. Many senior authors will let you "earn" first authorship – that is, they will not initially commit to having your name up front but if you perform the bulk of the work, will move you into this position. Unfortunately these discussions can become very fraught, particularly when your coauthor is your primary mentor. Complicating the issue, many textbook editors prefer or even require that the senior author's name be first, for pure name recognition purposes.

If this is your first chapter, your senior coauthor will need to mentor you through the project. Don't be afraid to admit this – mentoring is an expected part of the teaching environment for senior faculty.

The editor and publisher will supply guidelines. You may be given a sample chapter to use as an example. The guidelines will specify not only style but also length, number and type of illustrations, and style and number of references. Follow these guidelines! If a sample chapter has been supplied, read and reread it until the style and rhythm of the language are fixed in your brain. Do not supply a comprehensive 30 page manuscript, bristling with references, when the task at hand is to contribute a short chapter for a compact review text for medical students.

The proposed table of contents will give you additional insight as to the scope of the project and help you identify areas of potential overlap. If you notice a large overlap between your chapter and another chapter or chapters, by all means contact that author. Remember that it is the editor's job to integrate all of the material into a cohesive whole. You can make your job easier, however, by not straying into extraneous areas that are unlikely to make it into the finished book.

Avoid historical flourishes at the start, unless it is clear from the sample chapter that the editor wishes to include these. When I edited a textbook on Breast Diseases, I had to cut innumerable first paragraphs that detailed the history of breast surgery. Make every word count!

Researching your chapter may take you deep into material that you need to know but that does not belong in your chapter. This is particularly apt to happen if you are involved in project that is a bit peripheral to your previous publications. After you finish your chapter, consider whether this background information might be put into a review article for others in your specialty. Let me be clear: you *cannot* publish the same information twice. But you may have a significant body of information that will never make it into that first publication because it is not appropriate for inclusion.

Here is an example. When I was a junior faculty member, I spent a summer researching and writing a chapter on "Surgery and Anesthesia in Sickle Cell Disease" for a textbook for hematologists. As a surgeon, I had to delve deeply into the physiology, epidemiology, diagnosis, and treatment of the sickle cell diseases. This was important background information that I had to understand in order to more clearly convey the critical points of my assigned topic. It had no place in a textbook for specialists. I took this leftover material and crafted two related review articles to educate my fellow surgeons on the pathophysiology of these disorders and how it affects surgery and perioperative care (see Chapter 5 – Review Articles).

Articles for Peer-Reviewed Publications

The rest of this book deals primarily with articles written for peer-reviewed publications – usually called "journals" for short. Again, relatively early in your career you may be invited to contribute to a manuscript that is to be submitted to a journal. Your first such opportunity may arise because you have the energy, time, and enthusiasm needed to analyze some data (or study some clinical material) that your mentor has not had time to address; it may come out of your own research in a mentored lab; or, finally, you may initiate and complete a project on your own.

Journals are the primary forum for communicating new knowledge to your fellow professionals. Material may first be presented at national or international meetings, but until it appears in a peer-reviewed journal, it is not generally accessible to the wider community of scholars. Journal articles have a major advantage over book chapters because articles can be located through PubMed searches, and chapters (as yet) cannot. This advantage is starting to disappear as people increasingly turn to Internet search engines to retrieve information.

As previously mentioned, peer-reviewed publications in established journals are what count toward promotion and tenure. As you start your scholarly career, become familiar with the major journals in your field.

Choosing a journal. Your mentor should give you some guidance as to where to submit your manuscript. You need to understand the factors that influence that choice. First of all, the material must match the readership of the journal – generalist versus subspecialist. Second, the journal may be pre-determined, if the material is to be presented at a particular meeting (where submission of a manuscript is required). Beyond those obvious factors, journals are chosen based upon prestige, and prestige is quantitated, for better or worse, by several numbers.

The commonest number that you will hear quoted when journals are ranked is the "Impact Factor." The Impact Factor or IF of a journal is calculated as a ratio, based upon the total number of articles the journal published during a given year (denominator) with the total number of subsequent citations of those articles in other indexed journals in the numerator (http://wokinfo.com/essays/impact-factor/). Clearly the Impact Factor lags several years behind the actual performance of a journal because the citations take a year or two to appear. Journal editors, advertisers, professional societies, and promotions committees scrutinize the IF of the journal. Editors want to publish articles that are scientifically valid, that will appeal to their readership, and that will boost their IF.

The IF is not always the best way to judge a journal. By their very nature, some journals will never attain high impact factors yet publish extremely high quality material. Papers which are highly specialized may not be widely cited, and journals which are similarly narrow in focus may not attain high IF's. This is why a detailed knowledge of the journals in the field and their readership is important.

What about Open Access journals? Open Access journals are a category of publications which transfer the cost of publication to the author and make the journal freely available, gratis, over the Internet. Some granting agencies require that any subsequent publications be "open access," reasoning that the public has already paid for your research (through the grant) and should be able to read your paper free of charge. Researchers recognize this and build the cost of publication (which can be around $1000) into their grant applications. The Public Library of Science (PLOS) is arguably the most familiar and prestigious of these (https://www.plos.org/about/). Many subscription-model (that is, "standard") journals will allow a paper to be published as an "open access paper," if requested and required by the author and granting agency.

Unfortunately, open access journals have proliferated and some may have purely financial reasons for existence. These have been termed "predatory open access journals" (http://scholarlyoa.com/2012/11/30/criteria-for-determining-predatory-open-access-publishers-2nd-edition/). When a paper has been rejected by several big-name journals, it may be tempting to turn to one of these, particularly if you happen to receive an e-mail soliciting manuscript submission. Publication in one of these journals doesn't help you. Consult a medical librarian!

The factors that influence journal selection can be summarized thus:

- Audience – match the audience to the material
- Impact factor – go for the highest you can get
- PubMed – stick with journals that are indexed in PubMed
- Open Access or traditional – what are the requirements of your funding agency?

Overlapping Publications

Duplicate publication (see below) is just plain wrong. But it is not unusual to end up writing multiple papers, book chapters, or web-published articles on a focused area. As noted above, even early in your career you may accumulate far more material than is relevant to the specific manuscript at hand. As you advance in your chosen field, you will start to develop an area of expertise. One publication builds upon another. This is how you become known in a particular area.

Several common ways to publish (acceptably) in more than one format include:

- Publishing background material accumulated during research as a review article
- An invited summary "state of the art" paper in your area of expertise
- A web-based summary for lay (and other non-specialist) readers

Be sensitive to the balance between the "monster paper" and "salami-slicing." The monster paper is a manuscript bloated beyond all recognition by your desire to include everything you know about the field. Salami-slicing, the inverse problem, is a derogatory term applied to writers who take a single research project and derive multiple papers from it, by slicing the data one way or another. The "least publishable unit" is another derogatory term that is sometimes applied to this kind of writing. Don't do it.

What is duplicate publication? The International Committee of Medical Journal Editors gives this definition: "Duplicate publication is publication of a paper that overlaps substantially with one already published, without clear, visible reference to the previous publication" (http://www.icmje.org/recommendations/browse/publishing-and-editorial-issues/overlapping-publications.html). This is considered fundamentally wrong because editors and readers anticipate that a publication in the peer-reviewed literature reflects new knowledge. Duplicate publication is thus unfair to editors and readers, generally violates copyright law, and misuses a scarce resource (the available space in the peer-reviewed literature).

It does not matter if the publications are in two different languages, although previous publication in a language other than English will often be considered acceptable. In any questionable case, always send the complete information (including a copy of the previous publication or manuscript) to the second editor in your cover letter. If your original manuscript was published in a non-English journal with a limited readership, an editor may choose to consider an English version adapted for a different audience. The key here, as with conflict of interest, is full disclosure.

What is considered acceptable secondary publication? The ICMJE statement referenced above further outlines the circumstances under which secondary publication of the same material may be warranted. The three most important features are:

- Get approval from both editors up front
- Write the second publication for a different readership
- Cite the first publication in the second

In addition, it may be appropriate to publish a preliminary report and then a full report when all data are available or analyzed. An example of such a situation would be publication of results of a clinical therapeutic trial when five year, then ten year, and so on data might justify new publication. For further details on acceptable overlapping publications, see the complete statement.

Plagiarism and Fraudulent Publication

Unfortunately, it is necessary to say a few words about plagiarism and fraudulent publication. The International Committee of Medical Journal Editors provides a comprehensive definition of both on their website (http://www.icmje.org/recommendations/browse/publishing-and-editorial-issues/scientific-misconduct-expressions-of-concern-and-retraction.html). Both plagiarism and fraudulent publication are, quite simply, wrong.

Plagiarism consists of lifting blocks of text or information from one publication and using them in your manuscript. This is "cut and paste" gone bad. Be careful, be respectful of intellectual property rights, and follow the rules of attribution. Be aware that most journals now run software programs designed to ferret out instances of duplicate text between a submitted manuscript and published material and it is highly unlikely that your efforts will go unnoticed.

Self-plagiarism occurs when you simply cut and paste your own materials from one manuscript to another. Even if your "methods" are unchanged from previous experimental work, find a way to reword, adapt, or summarize (and cite previous work) instead of duplicating text.

Fraudulent publication occurs when data are fabricated, altered, or manipulated to influence the results. Sometimes people (unfortunately) do this deliberately. Such instances may be reported by co-workers, or suspected when the results are "too good to be true" or cannot be replicated. Papers that are found to be based upon fraudulent data are retracted by the journal in which they were published, with a very public statement.

There are more subtle ways in which data can be manipulated to shape the results. For example, suppose you are reporting on a small series of cases and have drawn certain conclusions. How should you handle new information, for example, a new case that alters your conclusions? What should you do if this information occurs after you have had an abstract accepted for publication but before you present your paper? These issues are beyond the scope of this brief publication, but are covered in more complete texts on research conduct (see Chapter 15).

The world of academic publication is a small one. The author who gets a reputation for plagiarism, fraudulent or duplicate publication is likely to find subsequent publication difficult if not impossible.

What about Publishing on the Internet?

Web publishing reaches a wider audience – generally both lay and professional. It allows a greater variety of ways to display and cite information, including hypertext, graphics, and videos. It is not unusual for published writers to put summaries of some of their material on their websites. Always cite the original publication and link to the PubMed citation. Do NOT simply paste the published paper onto your website; the copyright belongs to the journal, not to you.

Copyright issues aside, writing for the Internet is fundamentally different. The text needs to be shorter, and the material heavier in visual material. You can easily incorporate video clips. In many ways, it is the inverse of print publication. Thus Internet publication ideally complements (rather than competes) with print.

Chapter 3. Types of Journal Articles

Wei Chen MD

For most medical writers, a journal article will be the first full-blown piece of writing they will attempt. This chapter outlines the initial steps in writing such an article and describes the various types of papers and journals.

As you prepare to write, I recommend that you accumulate a file of examples of papers that you have found easy to read. These can be used as models for your own writing. This kind of model is paradoxically most useful when it deals with a topic different from your own, maybe even something that you are basically not interested in. Find a paper that captures your attention even if the topic is remote from your own field of endeavor.

For example, if you are writing a paper on a retrospective analysis of 100 cases of acute pancreatitis, a well-written paper on a retrospective analysis of 120 cases of leaking abdominal aortic aneurysms or 150 cases of blunt abdominal trauma might be useful. There is far less likelihood of inadvertent plagiarism if the topic is different from your own. Creative writers call this process "reading as a writer." Engineers call it "reverse engineering."

Next, consider your readers. Who are you trying to reach? Are your target readers emergency medicine physicians, or surgeons specializing in gender re-assignment? Identifying your target readers helps you determine what journals to which you will submit your paper. Think about the nature of the material you are going to write about. Are you describing the result of a multi-year translational research project? Are you reporting a rare disease? Or are you announcing a novel surgical technical breakthrough? Knowing the nature of your material allows you to decide what type of paper you are going to write. With this you can look up the specific requirements and instruction for the particular type of paper you are going to write from the individual journal websites.

To summarize, before you start to write, formulate a plan that includes your target readers, journals, the type of paper, and the specific requirements unique to these.

Now, on to the different types of papers. These are introduced here and then each considered in greater detail in the chapters that follow.

Case Reports

"What a great case! We should write it up!" How many times have I heard that from residents? My reaction is always mixed - I'm glad they want to write, but I also know it may be difficult to get case reports published. Case reports are not high on journal reviewers acceptance lists because only limited knowledge can be extracted from a single case. Having said that, don't let this discourage you. If you come across an interesting case that you consider worthwhile of publication, by all means write it up! An increasing number of journals specialize in case reports. Some of these are listed in Chapter 4.

Many medical advances/breakthroughs started out as case reports. For example, the supermicrosurgical lymphaticovenular anastomosis technique, now considered the state-of-the-art surgical treatment of lymphedema, started out as a non-English case report published in a Japanese journal. The total face transplant which recently contributed monumentally to our understanding of human allotransplantation also started as a case report.

The basic format of a case report is introduction, case presentation, and discussion. The introduction should indicate why you are writing this case up? What so special about it? What can I as a reader expect to learn from this?

To make your case report more interesting, include pictures. A case report describing a surgical technique would especially benefit from pictures. Pictures make your paper more engaging and interesting to the readers. When including pictures, use photo-editing programs to optimize the color and contrast, and to add annotation. Use these helpful editing tools to point out important anatomic structures. If you do not have any relevant pictures, draw them! Talk to a medical illustrator around you.

If a picture is worth a thousand words, what is a video worth? Yes, a video adds a lot of appeal to a paper, especially if it is a surgical paper. Imagine if you are writing a paper describing a novel surgical technique that is easy and effective. Is it more convincing to "say" that it is easy and effective or is it more convincing to "show" the readers in a video and let them come to that conclusion? Today, with the widespread use of smartphones and head-mount camcorders, recording a surgical video has never been easier.

Prior to shooting a picture/video, be sure to obtain proper consent from the patient. Let the patient know that the picture/video may be used for medical publishing purpose. Also be sure to protect the patient's privacy by blacking out identifying non-pertinent anatomic features.

Having illustrated your case with colorful pictures or a video, discuss your case. In the discussion the related current literature should be reviewed. Mention whether a similar case has been previously reported. The learning points in the case report should be elaborated to echo what was already said in the introduction. See Chapter 4 for more details about writing a case report, including detailed recommendations from some journals and a partial list of journals that actively solicit and publish this kind of paper.

Clinical Series

A clinical series is the logical extension of a case report. When you have encountered one interesting case, you can write it up as a case report. After you have encountered five or ten such cases, it may be time for a clinical series. A clinical series helps identify trends and patterns. It confirms and magnifies the significance of a finding initially reported in a case report. Everything that was said about a case report applies to the clinical series. In addition, the unifying features that tie these individual cases together into a series need to be thoroughly discussed. The findings in a clinical series do not need to be novel. In fact, these papers rarely contribute new information to the literature. They are nevertheless welcomed by the journals because they help solidify understanding of topics previously reported only in case reports.

In addition to summarizing the case series information in tabular format, it may be helpful to provide an in-depth description of two to four representative cases to further engage readers. Use pictures/illustrations/videos in these case examples. As said before, they speak a lot more to the readers than your words and tables. Always observe the requirements for informed consent and respect patient confidentiality.

Generally a clinical series follows the structure of a research paper. See Chapter 6 for more details on this, with details of each individual section.

Research Paper

This is the commonest type of paper in most journals. It is a report of original research, whether clinical, epidemiological, translational, or basic science. The standard elements include:

- Abstract
- Introductory paragraph
- Methods and Materials
- Results
- Discussion (with conclusions)
- References.

Detailed considerations for writing this type of paper are given in Chapter 6. This section is intended to provide an introduction.

The **abstract** may be either structured or unstructured depending on the journal. Refer to the journal you are interested in submitting to for specific requirements. A structured abstract has section titles for different parts of the abstract. An unstructured abstract does not. Structured or not, an abstract needs to contain the following elements – an introductory sentence stating why the study was performed, a brief description of the methodology, summary of the salient results, and concluding sentence or two giving the bottom line. The last sentence typically should answer the questions raised in the introductory sentence. Many readers will read only the title and the abstract - use the abstract to give the major points and to convince the reader to read further.

Moving on to the body of the paper, the **introductory paragraph** gives the background of the study. What question was the study designed to answer? What is currently known? Why is your study interesting (why did you do the study)? Keep this brief. An excessively long introduction is distracting and may cause the readers to lose interest. Get to the point and move on.

The **methods section** describes how the study was performed. This is where patient selection criteria, the study design, the duration of the study, how the patients were followed up, how the data were collected and how they were analyzed are discussed. This section needs to be sufficiently detailed that another researcher can replicate your study by reading this. If you are writing a surgical paper, describe your technique and the instruments used. Again, another surgeon needs to be able to

30

replicate your procedure by reading this (provided he/she is as good as you are). If the data analysis includes statistical calculations, then the statistical methods need to be described in detail. Involve your biostatistician in this.

Results may be presented in narrative, tabular, or graphic form; or a mixture of all three forms. Use tables and graphs efficiently to avoid being verbose in your narrative and also to make your results easily understandable. Consider the presentation of results from the readers' perspective. It should be clear, concise, and coherent. When done correctly, after reading the result section, the readers should come to a logical conclusion identical to yours.

The **discussion** puts the results in context and does not restate the results (a common error). This is the place to put more "flesh" in, to help the readers get a more in-depth understanding of your findings. This is also where your study is put in the context of the current knowledge of the topic. For example, if you created a new surgical technique that decreased the surgical time of a procedure to 2 hours, it would be relevant to point out that the average surgical time based on previous studies was 6 hours. Think from the reader's perspective. What questions would they have reading this? Working through this hypothetical series of questions will make your paper more satisfying and increase the chance of successful submission to journal. The questions need not be stated explicitly, but rather can be used as topics for paragraphs in the discussion.

Finally, conclude the paper powerfully by answering the questions raised in the introduction. After reading a well-crafted discussion, the majority of the readers should already agree with you. Drawing the conclusion should at this point be stating the obvious. Take care not to overstate the significance of your results, or to draw conclusions that are not supported by your results. This is not only wrong, but is a common reason cited in rejection letters.

The number of **references** should be appropriate to the journal, the topic, and the nature of the material. In most cases, 10-20 is a good range. Refer to each journal's instruction for authors and follow their guidelines.

Review Article

What do you do when you want to get an in-depth understanding of a complex topic in the shortest possible time? Many people turn to a review article to summarize current thinking on a topic. So keep that in mind when you write one. Such a paper is particularly appropriate, or may even be in demand, for controversial topics. The prerequisite of a high quality review paper is a thorough literature review. You know that you are ready to start writing when you find yourself so immersed in the topic that you start to talk to your friends and families about it.

Systematic reviews and meta-analyses are special types of research projects that result in review-type papers. See Chapter 5 for more information. Consider these if your paper will evaluate the results of a particular diagnostic or therapeutic intervention. The rest of this section refers to the ordinary type of review article, commonly written by beginners.

Begin with an introduction that sets the background for discussion. In the body of the paper, summarize the current state of knowledge, including studies that either support or conflict with each other. Having brought the readers up-to-date on the current literature, start a discussion. Here are some typical questions that a review article might address: How valid are the assertions made by the individual studies? What is the current standard of practice? Is there even a standard of practice? If not, what would it take to establish one? What are the future directions of research? Keep your discussion objective and impartial. Include a comprehensive (but not exhaustive) reference list.

Miscellaneous Publications

These include a wide variety of other venues such as CME papers, expert viewpoints, reply to a previously published paper, and letters to the editor. These papers are still peer-reviewed, but they are frequently subjected to less rigorous acceptance criteria. The specific format and content depends on the type of the paper. Since these papers usually do not involve a study, are short, and are relatively easier to write and to get accepted, they can be ideal projects for clinicians with busy practices. See Chapter 7 for more details. Now it's time to start writing!

Chapter 4. Case Reports

Alice M Fagin MD

Every time I give a lecture on medical writing, one or two young surgeons come up afterwards, eager to tell me about a "great case" they want to write up. They ask me where they should send their (proposed) case report. Unfortunately, my usual response has been, "Don't do it." I'm starting to rethink this response, because case reports (and the journals that publish them) are currently experiencing resurgence.

Almost every clinician starts their writing career with a case report. Case reports are easy to conceptualize – you have a great case, a real zebra, and your diagnostic and therapeutic acumen really shone. Several well-meaning people may even say, "You should write that up!" You put a lot of time and energy into your case report, but nobody seems to want to publish it. That's frustrating, and that is why you should think long and hard *before* you commit your time and energy to this kind of project.

This chapter will begin by defining a case report, and explaining why it is so hard to get a case report published. It will present the arguments *against* writing a case report. Then, for those of you who decide to push on, I'll give you the classic structure of a case report, tell you how to write a good case report, and provide a partial list of journals dedicated to the publication of case reports. Finally, I'll discuss alternative ways to publish the material you have gleaned during this fascinating case.

What IS a Case Report?

The CARE guidelines (http://www.ncbi.nlm.nih.gov/pmc/articles/PMC3844611/) define a case report as a "narrative that describes, for medical, scientific, or educational purposes, a medical problem experienced by one or more patients." It's a story about what you saw, did, or fixed, during the care of one specific patient.

At first glance, a case report appears to be simply an opportunity to show off your medical acumen. But it should be much more than that. At its best, a case report shows the medical community a rare or newly discovered medical issue/disease process/procedure. The number is too small for even a series of cases, let alone a prospective trial. The case is a true "zebra," but one that taught you a lot. Take that case, review the literature, explain the case, delve into the minutiae, research the important aspects, and write it up. That is a case report!

Why write one? Because they are short and highly focused, case reports take less time to write than other articles. Generally, the patient is one you have personally treated so the actual case description itself should already be written in your notes and in your head. If it is truly an uncommon process, then the available literature will be minimal and so your time researching on the computer will be limited.

More importantly, if your patient is truly that unique, then the medical community may benefit significantly from your experience. If the clinical situation is such that it cannot be reproduced (and thus rigorously studied), on purpose, for ethical reasons, your experience may prevent disasters for other providers. You may have just found the next HIV/AIDS epidemic in its infancy. Or you may have just stumbled upon the next big thing. You might, on the other hand, have a case which clearly illustrates the application of clinical guidelines toward a successful outcome. The journal "Clinical Case Reports" (http://onlinelibrary.wiley.com/journal/10.1002/(ISSN)2050-0904), one of several that welcomes case reports, is interested in common cases as well as rare ones. Other similar journals are listed later in this chapter.

Why NOT write one? First of all, realize that there is no real way to provide patient privacy and write a good case report. You *must* get the consent of the patient, and may wish to allow the patient to review the manuscript or even to add their perspective at the end. Check with your institutional officer to make sure that all of the necessary procedures have been followed.

Next, with the exception of "Clinical Case Reports" and some other journals noted at the end, it is very hard to get a case report published. Case reports suffer from the problems of applicability and generalizability. Whenever you read an article, you should ask yourself if the population studied is applicable to your patient population. This is very hard to do when the n is 1. If your patient is female, then men are out. If you are treating an elderly patient, your findings may not be applicable to a twenty-something or child. If your patient is Asian, Caucasian, African-American, or Hispanic, all the others may not experience the same situation or symptoms similarly. A case report, by its very nature, is specific to the single case being described.

Then there is the commitment to writing. In the world of not enough time to do everything I am supposed to do…you know, the world in which residents and junior faculty live…you need to choose where to expend your time and energy. If you write a paper that never gets published, you have just wasted valuable time. Many mainstream surgical journals do not publish case reports. Some of the specialty journals will still publish a select few but the report must contain something very special or out of the ordinary. Often, unknown to you, they have a large backlog of accepted case reports and may have imposed a moratorium on acceptance.

Consider your case – was it really that unique, or was it simply something you had never encountered? Get objective information by doing a literature search as well as by consulting senior colleagues.

Some specialties may be more amenable to publishing case reports than others. For example, an unusual presentation with striking imaging findings may find a home in a radiology journal, or a journal directed to emergency medicine practitioners. A case report that clearly illustrates the diagnosis and treatment of an unusual condition might be of interest to primary care providers. The work of seeking out a journal outside your normal discipline will require extra time and energy, and some journals will tacitly expect a co-author in their discipline.

There are always the "throw-away" journals – that is, heavily-illustrated free journals that depend upon advertising for revenue. These do not result in a PubMed citation and may not count toward promotion and tenure.

Journals that publish case reports, including case report specific journals, have gotten much more stringent with their requirements for publication. "The Journal for Medical Case Reports" (http://www.jmedicalcasereports.com/) states, to quote from their website, "Our aim is that every case report published in our journal will add valuable new information to the world's medical knowledge." Remember, journals get graded just like everyone else. Although other systems have been proposed, the dominant journal grading system remains the Impact Factor (http://wokinfo.com/essays/impact-factor/).

Authors are similarly graded! This means that journals only want to print that which will encourage further research and publishing. Case studies have historically not been cited much past their own publication so case reports tend to decrease a journal's impact factor by increasing the denominator without increasing the numerator. The case report has become a casualty of the pursuit of the impact factor.

Remember, too, that journals are not the only way you build a body of work in the medical world. If you are looking for podium time at a national conference, it is unlikely to be won with a case report. Most conferences are inundated with submissions and are looking for the same impact as journals. A case report might make the poster session at best.

Alternatives. Don't despair, there are alternatives to the case report and some take similarly little time. As stated before, maybe an aspect of your patient's care is worthy of publication. A striking image may be accepted on its own merits. An unusual electrocardiogram tracing, a photograph of a skin lesion, or a classic radiograph may be published. Some journals are always in search of images.

Try a letter to the editor of your favorite journal. If your patient's situation is that spectacular, then connect the patient's story with your letter. You never know, maybe your letter will prompt the request for more information and possibly a "case report on demand."

Other possibilities include designing larger trials. A retrospective review is a great place to start. Or try a case series or maybe even a cohort study. For the more computer-savvy, maybe a meta-analysis is the way to go. The point is that there are options, and almost any one of them is more likely to be published than a case report.

Why are Case Reports Significant?

I am definitely NOT trying to say that there is no room in literature for the case report. I, myself, am the author of published case reports. There are some things in medicine that just do not lend themselves to a randomized controlled trial. New or emerging medical conditions are best described in case reports. Case reports are helpful in identifying adverse or beneficial effects, recognizing new diseases, or explaining unusual presentations of common disease. For example, the relationship between thalidomide and congenital abnormalities was first described in a case report.

Clinical trials can dilute out or even lose the important detailed information about the patients because the results are aggregated. Case reports can help to elucidate interdependence of sequential events; variability in treatment schedules, dosages, and regimens; concomitant or causal comorbidities; contingency decision-making; and information missing from quantitative data.

Case reports have value, particularly with the increasing importance of individualized care. What is more individualized than focusing so much on a single patient that you do extensive research and tell others about the care for them to compare and contrast their own individual patients.

Additionally, with the emphasis of case-based learning in medical school, case reports may be an important aspect of future medical education. Case reports can guide individualization and personalization of treatments in clinical practice. The editors of the "British Medical Journal Case Reports" (http://casereports.bmj.com/) state that they want things that "are deemed of particular educational value. It is important that the learning outcomes of the articles are important and novel."

The other unique aspect of case reports is the ability to discuss medical mistakes. While no one wants to admit to mistakes, we all know that they do happen. A well written case report could possibly stop the same mistake from being made and save lives. We learn best through what NOT to do, and patients tacitly expect you to learn from others' mistakes rather than making them yourself.

Structure of a Case Report

In 2014, the Case Report (CARE) Group (http://www.ncbi.nlm.nih.gov/pmc/articles/PMC3844611/) put together guidelines for writing case reports. This had been done previously for other study designs and the group felt that guidelines could help smooth out the uneven quality of published case reports. The overall goals of developing guidelines was to "improve the completeness and transparency of published case reports and that the systematic aggregation of information from case reports will inform clinical study design, provide early signals of effectiveness and harms, and improve healthcare delivery." Their recommended components include:

- Title
- Keywords
- Abstract
- Introduction
- Patient Information
- Clinical findings
- Timeline
- Diagnostic assessment
- Therapeutic intervention
- Follow-up and outcomes
- Discussion
- Patient perspective
- Informed consent

We will discuss each aspect here. Note that *not all parts merit equal consideration* for any particular case.

As you prepare to write your case report, remember to keep your focus on the important and unique aspect of your case. Is it the presentation or the diagnosis? The management? The outcome? Or, maybe, the patient perspective? Always write with your key message in the forefront of your mind.

Each journal may want a slight variation on the theme, so pick a journal and check their website for specific instructions to the authors. And remember, brevity is part of a case report. Not all sections will deserve equal weight.

Title: Should include the words "case report" as well as the phenomenon of greatest interest, whether that is an aspect of the history, physical, test, or intervention. Avoid "teaser titles" such as "An Unusual Complication of…" in favor of greater specificity.

Keywords: Pretty self-explanatory. Think, "How do I want people to find my article in perpetuity?" Short, concise, 2-5 words. If possible, use MeSH headings (https://www.nlm.nih.gov/bsd/disted/meshtutorial/introduction/index.html).

Abstract: This should be your entire article, condensed. Start with what the case adds to medical literature. Add a shortened version of your patient presentation: *main* presentation, *main* clinical findings, *main* diagnoses and interventions, and *main* outcomes. In other words, think *"main."* Finish your abstract with your conclusion. What is your take home message?

Disclosure Statement: Have you received funds from any commercial entity? Do you have a financial stake in any corporations? For most young authors, the answer is "no." If you happen to be affiliated with any companies or products that might bias your conclusions, list these here. Full disclosure is the rule.

Introduction: Brief background summary of your reason for writing about this case. A few sentences should suffice. Reference the existing literature, if appropriate. If what you are describing is a new phenomenon, there may not *be* much literature out there. Try to find some common ground. Perhaps a similar, but not exactly the same, problem has been described. Or maybe there is evidence to support a different intervention, in which case you can contrast your findings with prior understanding. Why are you publishing this case report? What does it add to the body of knowledge?

Patient Information: This should be the real heart of the paper! At its most basic, a case report is a narrative, so give the reader a story to follow along with. Basic demographics are presented such as age, gender, race/ethnicity, occupation. As you write this section, consider what the basic message of your case report is going to be. If the take home message concerns a difficult diagnostic work-up, then the presentation and diagnosis are the most important part. If an intra-operative management decision or innovative technical modification saved the day, then careful description of this part becomes more important than the presenting symptoms

In any event, remember that you are telling a story. Make the reader see the patient as you first did. Explain how they presented, what the symptoms were, how they were affected. Then, keep us involved with their life and experiences with their medical, family, surgical, and psychosocial history. Include diet, lifestyle, and genetic information where relevant. Round out the picture with comorbidities and previous interventions/outcomes that may be significant with your own interaction. Help us to know your patient as well as you do.

Clinical Findings: Now you get your chance to add yourself into the story. What did you see, hear, feel, smell, even taste? What did that patient look like sitting or lying across from you? Describe the physical exam, but be selective. Summarize details that are not important to the take home message.

Timeline: This is a great opportunity for a diagram, table, or figure. Help us to understand, did this happen in 2 minutes or 2 months? Did it take a long time to determine the diagnosis but then a short time to treat or was it the other way around? Did the length of time needed affect the outcome? Give important dates and times to show how the key events of the case unfolded. Remember a great benefit of the case report is to show how a case unfolded, step by step. Think back to presentations that you have given or watched at various case conferences, such as Surgical Morbidity and Mortality, and you will understand how a slide illustrating the timeline of a complex case can facilitate understanding. Think about ICU flow sheets and diagrams. Imagine how clearly a timeline could illustrate the (failed) response to several drugs, then the successful response to the one that worked.

Diagnostic assessments: In this section you should discuss what diagnostic assessments you did. But, again, in narrative form, tell us why you did them, what complications or challenges they presented, other tests considered and why they were not pursued. Add prognostic characteristics, for example – tumor staging, when applicable. Sometimes the addition of cost data may be significant. If you were able to find a particularly cost-effective route to the final diagnosis and effective treatment, this information is important.

Therapeutic intervention: This is your moment to shine. Tell us what you did and how you saved the patient. Let us into your mind for a brief moment so that we may think as you think and see as you see. Explain why you did what you did and maybe why you changed course mid-stream. Give us your pro/con list and rationale. Explain dosages, strength, and/or duration of each intervention. For surgeons, innovative technical tips and tricks are always of interest. Photographs, line drawings, or video clips (for online journals) add immeasurable value.

Follow-up and outcomes: Explain what happened then…Tell us about adherence to your interventions. Explain what went well and what could have gone better. Fully discuss any adverse and unanticipated events; some of our best learning is done through failure. And here is another opportunity for pictures or images to show progression/regression/etc.

Discussion: If your patient information was the heart of the article, your discussion should be the brain. Delve deeply into the patient interaction. Explain the strengths and limitations of your management. Bring in the available literature to either corroborate what you did or so you can refute previous claims. Maybe explain how you used something that has previously been used but for a new purpose, a new diagnosis, or a new outcome. Explain your rationale again for what was done and why it worked or didn't work. Finish this section strong with your true "take away" lesson.

Patient perspective: If possible, this is a real strength of a case report. Large series or prospective trials cannot follow up with all the patients. Since you only have one patient, you can bring a unique perspective into the discussion, the perspective of the patient him or herself. We all read articles all the time telling us what we as doctors and surgeons think. We read literature and re-read articles agreeing or disagreeing but often the actual patient is lost. This is a wonderful opportunity to bring that patient back into the forefront of their own care. See how they feel about what happened and what was done with/to them. See if their opinion of the outcome matches yours. For some excellent examples, see the New England Journal of Medicine feature "Case Studies from the Massachusetts General Hospital," in which surviving patients often add a paragraph or two of "patient perspective" at the end.

Informed Consent: This can be a simple statement that the patient gave informed consent. Per CARE guidelines, consent becomes informed *when the patient or a relative reads the case report and approves its contents.* If the patient is deceased and no family is available you may need to get consent from an institutional committee. The best way to find this committee would be to contact your institution's Privacy Officer or Privacy Review Board. See specific "instructions for authors" for the journal you are submitting to.

Enhancing your Case Report

Many journals now only publish case reports on-line. A good way to increase the likelihood of publication is to have that unusual or interesting image, including a video clip. For example, I had an echocardiogram taken at diagnosis of Takotsubo cardiomyopathy and another taken at resolution. Obviously, this would not necessarily help in print but on-line the entire movie was able to be seen, ventricular ballooning and all.

Specifically for the surgical specialties, a great enhancer is to be able to describe and/or diagram your intervention. If people can follow what you did and are able to then replicate it, your case report has actually done some good.

Many doctors are very visual. We all are busy and have only so much time to devote to reading, often skimming, literature. Any additional visual that may catch the eye will increase the likelihood of your article being read, and even of your article being chosen for publication in the first place.

Respecting Confidentiality

Respecting your patient's confidentiality is an important aspect of your everyday care. Even with patient consent, do not include the name, initials, or medical record number. Carefully scrutinize any images. Do those numbers in the corner of the CT slice represent a patient identifier? Remove them.

Getting Permission from the Patient

For many years, this was overlooked. Since all identifiers were removed, there seemed little reason to ask for permission. But that was a mistake and one you should seek not to repeat. Explain to the patient, why you think the report should be written. Most people truly will want to help promote better care. Once you have treated the patient and developed a therapeutic relationship, gently bring in the idea of writing up their case. This is a great opportunity to also ask for them to write their own perspective. Follow all of your institutional guidelines and obtain informed consent from your patient.

Journals that Publish Case Reports

There are several ways to find a good journal that might be interested in publishing your case report. There is a specialized search engine called JANE or Journal/Author Name Estimator (http://www.biosemantics.org/jane/) that allows you to enter your abstract or title. JANE then suggests names of journals that have published similar papers. You can query PubMed (http://www.ncbi.nlm.nih.gov/pubmed) by putting "Journal of Case Reports in _____." (Insert specialty of your choice) into their search engine. Be aware that many of these are new, open access journals, and there may be a charge for "article processing."

Here is a short list of journals that specialize in case reports, with hyperlinks to their websites (as of October 2015). The list is meant to be representative, not exhaustive, and concentrates on journals that might publish case reports written by surgeons. Many other such journals exist. No endorsement of these particular journals is implied. Read the instructions to authors with care and speak with a medical librarian (if one is available).

- "Journal of Medical Case Reports" (http://www.jmedicalcasereports.com/)
- "American Journal of Case Reports" (http://www.amjcaserep.com/)
- "British Medical Journal Case Reports" (http://casereports.bmj.com/)
- "International Journal of Surgery Case Reports" (http://www.casereports.com/)
- "Journal of Surgical Case Reports" (http://jscr.oxfordjournals.org/)
- "International Medical Case Reports Journal" (http://www.dovepress.com/international-medical-case-reports-journal-journal)
- "Clinical Case Reports" (http://onlinelibrary.wiley.com/journal/10.1002/(ISSN)2050-0904)
- "Journal of Investigative Medicine High Impact Case Reports" (http://hic.sagepub.com/)
- "Case Reports in Critical Care" (http://www.hindawi.com/journals/cricc)
- "Clinics and Practice" (http://www.clinicsandpractice.org/index.php/cp)

Some journals will publish case reports of extraordinary significance as "Letters to the Editor." Another, less widely read alternative is a local journal, kind of a "home-grown" journal, from your institution. For example, the Department of Obstetrics and Gynecology at the University of Iowa houses an open-access peer-reviewed journal "Proceedings in Obstetrics and Gynecology" (http://ir.uiowa.edu/pog/). Most, but not all, of the articles in this journal originate at the University of Iowa. These are relatively rare, but are a great option if available at your institution. Don't overlook these if your article has been rejected by the bigger names.

Any or all of these alternatives generally count more in your Curriculum vitae than publication in a "throw-away" journal.

The Review Article as an Alternative to a Case Report

So, have I convinced you to write that case report, or not to write that case report? Whether your answer is "yes" or "no," I would like to recommend another option. A review article often doesn't take much more effort or time than a case report. A review article can pull together all of the (presumably scanty) information and previous case reports, use some of your images as illustrations, and allow you to go one step further with your discussion.

If you decide to follow this path, avoid including case details. A review article is not simply a disguised case report. Case details become irrelevant in the larger picture. This allows you to completely preserve patient confidentiality. The chapter that follows will tell you how to write a review article.

Chapter 5. Review Articles

Research is important, but review articles are valuable too. Busy clinicians love review articles. Editors love review articles as well, because they are popular with readers. Thus, good review articles are often-cited and frequently-downloaded, two key metrics for journal success.

Review articles may be divided into three general categories. First, there is the narrative review of a specific topic, written much as one might write a book chapter. We'll call this the "standard review paper" (or "review paper" for short) in this chapter. Then there are more specialized types – the "systematic review" and the "meta-analysis." These are really best thought of as research projects in and of themselves.   The bulk of this chapter will deal with the standard review article, and the end of the chapter will provide an introduction (and links to some handy resources) to the other two forms.

There are two general circumstances in which you might write a standard review article. For some neophytes, it is the very first paper that they are asked to write. For example you might have done a great job of presenting a topic at Grand Rounds and either you or your mentor, or someone in the audience, suggests "writing this up." Or you have chosen to write up a case report or a cluster of cases as a review article as recommended in Chapter 4. Where to start? This chapter is aimed at you.

The second situation arises when you have a body of published work in a specific area and you are invited to (or decide to) write a paper summarizing the state of the art. By this time, you are a fairly accomplished author and only need a bit of additional guidance.

Writing Your First Standard Review Paper

Do your research. Make sure that the topic you have selected will be of interest to readers (ask some colleagues), that it has not recently been covered in a review paper in a major journal, and that it is sufficiently important to merit your time.

Consider whether your topic might be amenable to the more stringent, but ultimately more valuable, form of review called a "systematic review." Systematic reviews are designed to look at all the available good data and answer a question, such as which intervention is better. It is a kind of hypothesis-driven project. It is possible that, as you delve into the literature, you might decide to do a systematic review. If so, follow the guidelines in the section at the end of the chapter. Make sure that you separate out the references (studies) that will be included in your systematic review from your more general initial literature search. Consult a medical reference librarian if in doubt!

Define the scope of the review. It is far easier to write a paper on a well-focused topic than to write one on something broad. Let's suppose that your hospital has a world-famous clinic specializing in sickle cell anemia and that you have had to become familiar with surgical disorders unique to this patient population, as well as their special needs during the perioperative period. Or maybe you just encountered your first case and managed it successfully.

You have noticed that there are no recent review articles in this area, and think that other surgeons might find a summary of the topic useful. Try to imagine the title of your proposed paper. If you find yourself considering two titles, "Surgical Conditions Associated with Sickle Cell Anemia" and "Perioperative Management of patients with Sickle Cell Anemia," then maybe you really should write two papers. Choose one, and get started. Keep a file for the second one and put ideas and articles into it as you go along.

Identify the intended audience. As you define the scope of the review, imagine the intended audience. Who will want to read this? Who needs to know this information? Are you going to submit your paper to a surgical journal? Or are you interested in educating hematologists about how surgeons treat various problems? Remember, that you may decide to choose your audience as you go along or after receiving several rejections.

Consider where you will submit the paper. Browse through several copies of a selection of journals that reach your proposed audience. Look at general style, tone, and how often each publishes review articles. Pick one and follow their requirements exactly. List your primary choice and a couple of fallback choices in your manuscript log (see Chapter 14) so that you do not need to repeat this process if the paper is rejected.

Review the literature. You probably have already done a comprehensive literature review. Repeat it, to see if anything new has been published. The ideal topic for a review article would, naturally, be something that is of general interest but that has not been reviewed recently. What does "recently" mean? It depends upon the topic and how fast it is evolving. If an area is developing rapidly, there may be a role for frequent updates. If nothing new has happened in an area, on the other hand, you will want to make sure there have not been any reviews published in the last 5 years or so.

If you have access to a medical library, enlist the help of a reference librarian. These individuals can help you refine your search and, in the process, teach you invaluable skills. They can also show you how to input references directly into a database from which you can eventually construct your reference list. Take advantage of their expertise.

As you read through your references, natural subtopics for your article will suggest themselves. Start listing these. Group your references into these subheadings.

Structure of a review paper. Check the specifications of the journal to which you are submitting. Most journals will want an abstract and all will want keywords. Start the bulk of your text with an introductory paragraph stating why you chose to review the topic and why the reader should read on. Identify your major subtopics and find a natural order in which to place them. Thus, if your topic is a particular disease, a natural order would be:

- (History) – optional
- Epidemiology
- Pathogenesis
- Diagnosis
- Treatment

In the hypothetical case of "Surgical Conditions Associated with Sickle Cell Anemia" a possible order might be:

- Brief introduction to sickle cell anemia
- List of specific surgical conditions, from most common to least common. Include diagnostic workup and treatment for each.
- Nonsurgical conditions that can mimic surgical problems

A paper on "Perioperative Management of Patients with Sickle Cell Anemia" might include sections on:

- Brief introduction to sickle cell anemia
- Medications used to treat the condition
- Optimizing preoperative status
- Anesthetic considerations
- Unique postoperative complications in this population of patients
- Minimizing postoperative complications
- Management of complications in these patients

Use major headings for each topic, and divide your manuscript into appropriate sized segments. Subheadings may be useful if a topic is particularly complex. There is no requirement that each topic receives an equal number of paragraphs (for example) but it is generally good to avoid extremely short or extremely long segments.

If you find that you have an extremely long segment with multiple subheadings perhaps that should be the focus of your paper. Extremely short segments may be included under larger topics. The primary criterion should be easy of reading.

Incorporating case material. By all means use specific case material (radiographs, histology, pathology) to illustrate your paper, if appropriate. Do NOT include any details of the case, however fascinating these may be to you. Simply include the image with a brief figure legend such as "Chest x-ray showing acute chest syndrome in a postoperative adult with sickle cell anemia. Note findings ____, ____, and ____." Editors will often reject out of hand any disguised attempt at getting a case report into the literature. Focus on the topic, not the case.

Make sure that the patient cannot be identified. Remove the name, medical record number, institution, and so on from any images.

Remember that you must not include protected health information without explicit permission from the patient. Check with the compliance officer at your institution if you have any questions. Be sensitive to the possibility that the patient or a relative may happen across your published report. If in doubt, always get consent from the patient!

Tables, lists, and algorithms. Consider incorporating tables or lists (for example, a list of complications encountered with sickle cell disease. If you are dealing with diagnosis or management, an algorithm summarizing a suggested pathway is ideal.

What about data? You may wish to include a table summarizing the key findings of several published series. Such a table may include, if appropriate your own published institutional experience.

Be careful about including your own unpublished data. Remember, a review article is not a research paper. Data deserves careful analysis and publication as a research paper, so that the methodology and findings can be thoroughly explained. Inclusion of unpublished data is thus inappropriate and may preclude subsequent submission of a research paper based upon your findings.

If the focus of your review is to critically compare and contrast published material on the topic, consider doing a systematic review or even a meta-analysis. These are generally more valuable contributions to the literature.

Adapting a review paper to a different audience. If you have written a review paper and cannot get it published in the specialty field of your choice, consider adapting the material for a different audience. Thus, a review of "Workup of the Patient with Bloody Nipple Discharge" may be rejected by surgical, breast, or oncologic journals as too basic. A Family Medicine or OB-GYN journal might find it extremely topical and eminently publishable. Always consider your message and your audience. Who else might benefit from your message?

Systematic Review

A systematic review is really a research project where the data comes from combining previously-published studies. As such, it has more of the structure of a research report (with methods, results, and discussion sections) than a standard review article. It does take more work to do a systematic review, but the end result may be a significantly more important contribution to the medical literature.

Systematic reviews generally deal with the results of particular interventions in specific patient populations. Thus, not all topics are amenable to the systematic review process. The acronym PICOS (Participants, Interventions, Comparisons, Outcomes, and Study design) summarizes the key features that are typically included in the objectives of such a review. If your topic does not deal with the first four, it is not worth performing a systematic review.

Thus, not all topics are amenable to systematic review. A topic such as "Prevention of adhesions in gynecological surgery" could definitely be addressed by systematic review (and has been). On the other hand, a general review of "The pathogenesis of breast abscesses," while potentially valuable and interesting, could not. The topic typically needs to deal with a specific diagnostic or therapeutic intervention and the outcomes of that intervention.

To perform a systematic review, first carefully define the research question, the characteristics of the population in which it is being studied, and how published material will be accessed. Because a careful electronic search strategy is integral to this kind of research, enlist the help of an experienced reference librarian. Be prepared to detail your search strategy in the methods section of your manuscript. The PRISMA checklist (http://www.prisma-statement.org/2.1.2 - PRISMA 2009 Checklist.pdf) provides a great summary of the key elements of a systematic review. It also provides a structure that you can follow as your write your manuscript.

The Cochrane Collaborative maintains a database of systematic reviews. If you are interested in preparing a systematic review for submission for publication and inclusion in their database, see their guidelines, available from http://www.cochranelibrary.com/help/how-to-prepare-a-cochrane-review.html.

Meta-Analysis

A meta-analysis takes the systematic review process one step farther. This is a very specific research project, beyond the scope of this introductory manual. By combining the results of multiple randomized clinical trials, a larger pool of data is created from which important conclusions may be drawn. Obviously, extreme care must be taken in defining how studies are chosen for inclusion or exclusion, and then statistically combined and analyzed.

A meta-analysis typically includes a systematic review, but goes far beyond it in scope and conclusions. The Cochrane Collaborative offers a comprehensive handbook (http://handbook.cochrane.org/) covering both systematic reviews and meta-analyses.

Chapter 6. Reports of Original Research

Scott Sherman MD

The bulk of material printed in medical journals consists of reports of original research. These include laboratory (also called bench or basic science) research, clinical investigation, translational research (that is, research which applies or translates basic research to the clinical setting), meta-analyses, and epidemiologic research.

In the general category of clinical investigation, studies vary in cost and complexity from multi-institutional prospective randomized clinical trials, through prospective non-randomized trials, all the way down to retrospective case collections. While the gold standard for strength of evidence remains the prospective randomized clinical trial, preliminary information gathered from retrospective and prospective studies often provides the initial data that propel the design and completion of a prospective randomized trial. In particular, many of the advances in surgery were made without randomized prospective trials.

This chapter will first describe the standard elements of any research report, and then describe strategies for actually tackling the writing. It is written for the absolute beginner, and intended to give a practical approach that will yield maximal results. Nothing can substitute for good mentorship, but even the most nurturing mentor will expect you to generate a rough draft on your own.

Tackling the Task

Always start with the end in mind. Identify your "target journal" – the journal to which you intend to submit the manuscript. To find a good target journal, look for articles on topics related to your manuscript, which use similar methodology and that are aimed at a similar readership . Access representative copies of that journal and refer to them throughout your writing process. Check the journal website for "Instructions for Authors." You will often find very detailed and extremely helpful suggestions.

Find some excellent, well-written examples of papers similar to your manuscript. You should already have created a file of model articles (see Chapter 3) – articles in fields of endeavor remote from your own, but clear and well-written and similar to the sort of research that you are doing. For example, if you are a colorectal surgeon, papers in the breast surgery or vascular surgery literature might serve as good models. For a vascular surgeon, papers from surgical oncology might fulfill this role. Avoid using articles in your own narrow field to prevent unconscious plagiarism.

Read through this entire chapter and formulate a plan of attack. Are you the sort of person who will want to start at the beginning and work through the manuscript section by section, or would you find it easier to tackle the sections out of order? Assemble all of your materials and get to it. Set yourself a goal of providing a draft to your senior author or mentor by a certain date, well in advance of your target date for final submission. Allow plenty of time for your mentor to respond.   Don't be afraid to show your draft to experienced writers in your department. The input of non-specialists may be extremely helpful, particularly if you plan to submit your paper to a journal that has a broad readership.

Additional hints on how to actually tackle any writing project are given in Chapter 8, and the mechanics of the final submission process are detailed in Chapter 9

Standard Elements

Each part of the manuscript has a specific role to play. A well-written manuscript tells a story that leads the reader through a process of discovery that imparts new knowledge. The standard elements include:

- Title
- Abstract
- Keywords
- Disclosure statement (including funding sources)
- Introductory material (also called "Background")
- Methods and materials (also called "Patients and methods")
- Results
- Discussion
- Conclusion or summary
- References

Most journals require that reports of clinical trial results adhere to the CONSORT (Consolidated Standards of Reporting Trials) guidelines. Their website (http://www.consort-statement.org/) offers a checklist, flow diagram, examples, and many other helpful items. Failure to comply may result in automatic rejection; conversely, using the CONSORT material will help to strengthen your manuscript. I strongly recommend that you refer to this material during study design and analysis, as well as during the final writing process. You will, of course, also need institutional review board (IRB) approval for any human studies; and similar approval for animal studies. All of this must be done before doing your actual research and then documented in your manuscript.

Title. The title should simply and concisely represent the contents of the paper. It helps readers retrieve your paper during a PubMed search, and it makes it easy for subscribers to decide if your paper is of interest or applicability as they scan the journal's Table of Contents. Avoid a "teaser" title such as "An Unusual Complication of ____" in favor of a more specific one such as "Portal Vein Thrombosis Following ____." Similarly, it is generally advisable to avoid claims of primacy. Titles such as "First report of…" simply invite a flurry of counterclaims of previous reports, often in journals not easily accessed through a PubMed search.

The ideal title gives both the topic and the major findings of the study. The title should be no more than one sentence long, and need not be a complete sentence. Subtitles are commonly used. Because the title may be lengthy, many journals also require a short "running title" that will be used as a header. If you only had five seconds to tell someone what your paper is about, what would you say? This is the nucleus of your title. The reader must be motivated by your title to look at your Abstract, which is the next section.

Abstract. If the title gets your foot in the door, the abstract is your opportunity to convince the reader that your paper is worth reading. Most journals require that you follow a standard structured abstract format. If you have submitted your material for presentation, it is likely you have already prepared an abstract and the temptation will be strong to simply paste that abstract into the appropriate space in your manuscript. While this may be a good initial strategy, it is important to realize that that abstract was written for a different purpose and to different specifications than the abstract that accompanies your manuscript. Carefully review the journal instructions to authors, and reconsider your abstract in its new role as an introductory summary before doing this. Word counts may be significantly different. Finally, an abstract submitted to a meeting may include tables or graphs, but these are generally not used in the abstract that introduces a manuscript.

Note that the abstract is generally retrievable through a PubMed search but that the manuscript may be only available to subscribers or through medical libraries. At best, the abstract is the part that may lead them to read your entire paper. At worst, it may be the only part of your manuscript that they read.

The standard elements of a structured abstract mirror the elements of the paper itself. Because the total number of words is limited, reserve the bulk of your abstract for your results and conclusions section. Even if the journal does not require a specific format, conceptualizing your abstract in these four sections will help you draft something effective. Make sure that every word counts and eliminate extraneous material. These are the standard elements, with some variation from journal to journal.

- **Background** – a single sentence explaining why you did the study. Why should the reader be interested? Why is this problem important or unresolved?

- **Methods** – this can be as brief as "A prospective observational cohort study was conducted." or "An analysis of a prospectively maintained database of ___ procedures from _____ to _____ was conducted." For some journals, a sentence fragment such as "Prospective observational cohort study" may be completely acceptable. If you are unsure, go through previous issues of the journal and note the style employed in presenting studies of similar experimental design.

- **Results** – here you enumerate your key findings, including specific numbers and p-values. Prioritize the information included here, and summarize less important results. For example, a simple sentence such as "the two groups were well-matched for age, sex, and comorbidities" will suffice. Concentrate on the key findings of your paper. If you were forced to list the top three findings, what would you say? You will give full details in the results section of the paper. Generally this is the largest section of the abstract, but even so, space is limited.

- **Conclusions** – This is the opportunity for you to make the case for your study. What does your data add to the body of knowledge about this condition and its management? Typically two or three sentences give the reader the most important messages. Avoid over-statement or hyperbole. It is easy to get carried away by your own enthusiasm. Remember that a common criticism of submitted manuscripts is "conclusions not supported by results."
- If you are reporting a clinical trial, many journals will require you to put the **trial registration #** at the end of the abstract, after the first use of the acronym representing the trial, or both.

Almost inevitably your draft abstract will be too long. There are two ways to shorten it: revision for brevity, and selective deletion of details. Always strive for economy of language. Strunk & White's classic book "The Elements of Style" is an excellent guide. Read (or reread) this book as you write the abstract and, subsequently, the entire manuscript. If you are within 20 or 30 words of your target word count, revision for *brevity* will generally take you to goal. If the abstract is twice as long as allowed, you may need to *selectively delete* less important details. Remember that the abstract is not only a summary of your most important findings, but also leads into your complete paper, where you will enumerate in complete detail all of the findings of your study.

A few journals use a very short summary in their Table of Contents, in addition to the standard abstract which is part of the paper. If so, the journal will give you specifications for this. Typically it consists of several sentences – the first stating the problem, and the rest giving major findings of the study (often without numbers or p-values).

Keywords. Most journals request 8-10 keywords. These help categorize your article and facilitate retrieval by readers searching PubMed and other databases. Keywords do not need to consist of single words. For example, "Breast cancer" is a keyword that consists of a two-word phrase. Most writers prefer to do the keywords last, because it often becomes obvious which words and phrases recur commonly and form themes in the manuscript. What keywords did you use when doing your literature search? These should form the nucleus of your 8-10 keyword list. If you are struggling, the input of your medical librarian may be helpful. MeSH (Medical Subject Headings) is a thesaurus maintained by the National Library of Medicine (https://www.nlm.nih.gov/mesh/). This set of standard terms facilitates searching within the National Library of Medicine databases. Terms are arranged in a logical twelve-level hierarchical structure. It is always best to use the most specific terms applicable. When an author assigns keywords that correspond to MeSH terms, accurate placement within this structure is facilitated. The MeSH homepage includes a searchable database of these terms.

Finally, some keywords are standard, global, and so obvious that you might overlook them. These might include "surgery," "surgical complications," and "infection." Use these to complete your keyword list, if you have exhausted more precise descriptors. If you are struggling to find enough keywords, think globally.

Background or Introduction. This is the first section of the manuscript. Some journals will have you label it as such, but in most this section, unlabeled, simply follows the abstract and begins the body of the text. Either way, this part makes the case for your work. Why did you do the study? Why should the reader care? In some journals, it may be as brief as two or three sentences. In others, it may extend to two to three paragraphs. Journal style definitely factors into your decision as to length. Resist the temptation to include a lot of historical information, unless this is strictly relevant. This material may or may not be appropriate for the discussion. Imagine you are trying to explain *why* you did the study to an interested colleague.

Strive to strike a balance between basic information and details. Often the first sentence or two of a draft can be eliminated. A sentence such as, "Breast cancer is one of the commonest causes of death of American women," really adds nothing new for most purposes. Ask yourself if this is information that essentially all of your readers already know – if so, eliminate it. Some writing instructors call this unnecessary preliminary verbiage "throat-clearing."

Methods and Materials. The title of this section varies with the topic of the paper. A common variant is "Patients and

Methods." Here you describe, as clearly as possibly, the methodology that you used. A knowledgeable reader should be able to replicate your study from the information included. For brevity, you may cite a standard methodology (with appropriate reference) rather than detailing it. A sentence such as: "_____ was measured using liquid chromatographic analysis as described by _____ (citation)" gives the necessary information without unnecessary detail. Make sure that the reference you cite actually clearly details the technique. This is also a good way to handle subsequent publications from your laboratory using the same methods.

Often a flow diagram showing the trial design with number of patients in subgroups provides the best representation, particularly in complex clinical trials.
Include details of your trial design and statistical analysis. Expert statistical review is a real plus, and you should cite and acknowledge your biostatistician.

In some cases, supporting details (such a questionnaire) may be included in an Appendix, rather than taking up space within the body of the manuscript. This material may or may not end up in the published paper, or may be available on the journal website – let the editor make that decision.

Results. Present your findings clearly and objectively. Avoid drawing any conclusions – save that for the Discussion section. As the investigator in the old television series Dragnet used to say, "Just the facts, ma'am." Although theoretically you could probably present all of your results in a series of tables or graphs with minimal narrative text, in practice the reader should be led through your results by text supplemented by graphs and tables when appropriate. If you go through your favorite journals, you will see that well-written papers strike a comfortable balance, including some text and some tables or graphs.

Begin with what might be considered "background data" – if you are reporting a clinical study, basics such as how many patients were included, as well as their age, sex, demographics, and other relevant material such as comorbidities may be discussed, or conveniently given in a table. After briefly establishing who or what was studied, the results of those studies must be digested into individual experiments or comparisons which are then reported in a sequence that makes sense. A results section best engages the reader by telling the story of an interesting question and the steps leading to its answer.

Before starting to write, it can be helpful to write down the overarching question of the study and the conclusion reached. Then, break the overall question into sub-questions with sub-answers. Ultimately, this should outline the specific experiments or comparisons that were conducted, and by organizing these in logical sequence, individual results paragraphs are created.

For each paragraph, an introductory sentence frames the question at hand, the body of the paragraph reports the results, and a concluding sentence concisely summarizes the key findings while linking them to the next experiment or investigation. A good strategy is to proceed from more general questions to the specifics, with each result answering one question and suggesting the next, which is then elaborated upon and answered in the following paragraph.

For presenting data, here are some general guidelines that I have found helpful:

- Comparison of a large number of variables between two or more groups where actual numeric values are of potential interest – use a table (example – laboratory values in two groups of patients)
- Comparison of selected variables between two (or more groups) where relative effect is more important than numeric value – use bar charts with error bars (example – laboratory values in experimental animals or cell culture)
- Comparison of variables where the degree of clustering or dispersion of data is important – use scatter plots with a regression line.
- Time trends of variables – use a graph with time on the x-axis, and the parameter of interest on the y-axis (example – weight loss after bariatric surgery over time)
- Survival data – use a Kaplan-Meier plot (example – cancer patient survival)
- Results of meta-analysis – use Forest (also sometimes termed Forrest) plots

Avoid duplication – do not state numeric results within the text and then refer to a table or graph showing the same results. Often tables will include a more complete listing of numbers, groups, or comparisons, while the text serves to further highlight and explain the one or two most important results, rather than restating the table in narrative form. Consider using subheadings if your results fall into natural groups. These subheadings can then be replicated in your Discussion section.

In the text of the Results section, you should also explain any exceptions and how they were handled. Were any patients lost to follow up? Were any cases excluded for any reason? Were there any outliers that might skew the data?

Try several ways of displaying your data and determine which format is the easiest to understand. Look through your file of model papers to see how experienced medical writers have handled this problem. If you are going to use graphs, photographs, or line drawings, make sure that your images correspond to the technical specifications of the journal. Most journals can now accommodate color images, but it is always wise to check because a few still charge the author for color reproduction.

Do not imbed graphs, charts, or images in the text of your manuscript. Follow the instructions of the journal and put these at the end. If you are going to create your own graphs, make sure these are clean and clear. Avoid the temptation to use 3-D effects in graphs unless it adds informational content.

Read Tufte's classic text "The Visual Display of Quantitative Information," referenced at the end, to understand how your images can add clarity or confusion.

Finally, explain how the data were analyzed (statistical techniques) and acknowledge your statistical consultant.

Discussion. This section explains the major findings of your study and puts your results into context. Usually this is the longest section of the paper. Consider this your opportunity to explain to the reader what questions you have answered and why those answers matter. It also allows you to address alternative explanations of your results, explain why your interpretation is correct, acknowledge limitations, and highlight avenues for future work.

Beginning writers often simply recapitulate the results, or conversely draw conclusions in the results section. To avoid this, as you write the discussion, keep the following questions in mind:

- **What are the primary findings of my study?** Remember that because of your intimate involvement with your work, the meaning and future implications of your results section might seem obvious to you, but they often are not to a first-time reader. Beginning the discussion by synthesizing the essential points of your primary findings (in different words) helps the reader understand your results and see them as you do. Then you must lead the reader with clear explanations down a path towards your interpretation of these results.

- **How does this confirm or contradict other studies?** If your study confirms other work, why is another study needed? Always explain how your work fits into a larger body of work on the topic. If your study contradicts other studies, you also need to explain why your work is important. At the same time, explaining discrepancies (methods, sample, changes in practice patterns) between your work and prior studies can also help you demonstrate how your findings add to the literature. Avoid critiquing the work of others; it is always possible that one of those authors will be a reviewer for your paper! Instead, emphasize how differences in study design/patient population/inclusion criteria set your work and results apart and how that makes your contribution valuable and unique.

- **What are the limitations of this study?** Acknowledge these frankly. Hoping that the reviewer will not notice any methodological limitations is generally futile, but by seizing the opportunity to provide your own explanation and justification for admitted weaknesses, you can promote your study's good points and preempt many potential criticisms. Openly address your study's faults, but do not strike too negative a tone or include excessive apology for your work's shortcomings. No study is perfect, and seen in another light, limitations also represent opportunities for future studies!

- **What new questions does your study raise or leave unanswered?** Your discussion should begin by explaining the most important and best-supported conclusions of your work. Later in the discussion, and perhaps combined with your acknowledgement of limitations, you may include limited speculation on implications of your research beyond what you have proven to be true. When doing this, be sure to not reach too far beyond your results and support your claims with other evidence when possible. (Good: "We have shown that chemical X inhibits growth of cancer cells in culture. Other groups have shown that chemical X downregulates BRAF signaling in the Map-kinase pathway, [citation] suggesting BRAF inhibition as a potential mechanism for chemical X's effects. Examining activation of BRAF and its downstream targets by western blotting after treatment with chemical X could help determine whether the observed growth inhibition in these cancer cells is indeed related to BRAF signaling." Bad: "We have shown that chemical X inhibits growth of cancer cells in culture, and thus the problem of human cancer is now solved.") Remember that any hypotheses you propose appear more plausible when you are able to suggest reasonable studies to test them in future work.

Finally, resist the temptation to delve into side issues. In the course of your literature search, you may very well have uncovered some fascinating information about the history of your topic, how it has been managed in the past, complications, and so on. All of this may be significant, but is it relevant? Save all of the material that you don't use – notes, references, and so on. As you continue to work and write in this area, the material that you accumulated may be used for other purposes. If nothing else, this extra material may provide the nucleus of a subsequent review article.

Use subheadings if necessary. If you used subheadings in your Results section, consider using the same subheadings in your Discussion.

Summary (Conclusions). This is the last paragraph of the discussion section, which allows you to very briefly restate your findings and major conclusions. Some journals will have you set it off as a separate section, and others will not. If the journal does not allow you a separate section, you may simply begin the first sentence of this final paragraph, "In conclusion, we found…" or some variation.

Although the discussion section allows some latitude regarding interpretation of your research, in the summary, be very careful to include only conclusions that your data firmly support.

When approaching this section, consider the key points you would like the reader to take away from your manuscript. Remember that some readers will have skipped ahead to the end without carefully reading the entire paper. Even careful readers will likely retain best what they read last.

References. How many references should you cite? Sometimes it is hard to know how many is just enough. For most papers in most journals, 10-15 carefully selected references will suffice, although these limitations are diminishing with electronic publication. You will have done a literature search when you embarked upon your project; take care to update your search at least two more times. Update it for the first time when you sit down to write the discussion. Update it again before you actually submit the manuscript for publication, and incorporate any new information into your discussion. If you find yourself with too many references, give priority to the most recent ones and those with the highest level of evidence. Make sure that you include recent references by others doing major work in this area; one of these individuals may be called upon to review your paper!

Use reference-managing software, so that you can easily insert and remove references and move them around in your manuscript as the discussion evolves. Many word processing programs incorporate this into their software. Most medical journals require that you list references in the order cited in the text, which means that if you change your discussion or add or delete a reference, you will need to renumber. While most journals use a standard PubMed reference format, there are minor variations from journal to journal. Reference-managing software will automatically renumber your references, and can help you change the format if you resubmit the completed (but, alas, rejected) manuscript to another journal.

CME/MOC Questions

If your article is accepted for publication and is sufficiently noteworthy, the editors may ask you to send several multiple choice questions for continuing medical education (CME) or maintenance of certification (MOC). This is usually not part of the initial submission process. If you are asked for these, see Chapter 7 for some tips on writing good questions. Don't worry about this during your initial writing process, unless the journal specifically requests these up front.

How to Tackle the Actual Writing

Where to start? Some people start by opening a new document, starting with the title page, and proceeding through the sections in order. Most of us find that completely blank document daunting and need to find a starting point. Start wherever you find it easy to begin. Let the momentum and enthusiasm you generate from that writing to carry you into the more difficult sections. Many writers begin with the Methods and Results sections, because these are the easiest to write, and do the Discussion last.

Melina Kibbe (see references) advocates starting with the Charts and Figures, then going through Methods and Results. She suggests that you then write the introductory material followed by the Discussion. In essence, this encourages you to write the manuscript as if you were telling a story. Find a method that works for you.

Chapter 8 gives more tips on the mechanics of getting the job done, regardless of the type of paper you are writing. This includes other aspects common to all manuscripts, such as the cover letter. Chapter 9 deals with the process of actually submitting your manuscript. Finally, Chapter 10 includes tips on revision after reviewers' critiques.

References and Resources

Browner WS. "Publishing & Presenting Clinical Research." 3rd edition. 2012. Philadelphia, PA. Lippincott Williams & Wilkins. This comprehensive text deals deals with all aspects of publishing clinical research. It also includes information about submitting abstracts to meetings, creating posters, and giving presentations.

Kibbe ME. Chapter 10. How to Write and Revise a Manuscript for Peer-Review Publication. In: Chen H and Kao LS (eds) "Success in Academic Surgery Part 1." 2012. London, Springer Verlag. This is an excellent resource with a lot of information about all aspects of an academic career.

Kibbe MR, Sarr MG, Livingston EH, et al. The Art and Science of Publishing: Reflections from Editors of Surgery Journals. Journal of Surgical Research. 2014 Jan;186(1):7-15. Recent presidential address from the Association for Academic Surgery presents results of a membership survey and gives cogent advice on various topics referable to publishing.

Strunk W Jr, White EB. "The Elements of Style."1959. New York, The Macmillan Company. This classic is worth reading and re-reading. It is available as an e-book at minimal cost. Even if you read this in college, go back and read it again.

Tufte ER. "The Visual Display of Quantitative Information." 2001. Connecticut. Graphics Press. This is a classic and elegant text that explains how graphs and other images can represent and clarify, or misrepresent and confuse, information. It is a delight to read.

Chapter 7. Special Forms of Articles

This chapter deals with various kinds of articles that don't precisely fit under the general categories previously discussed. Invited contributions are covered first. The end of the chapter addresses some miscellaneous types of short writing, such as editorials and documents for continuing medical education events.

Invited Contributions

Paradoxically, an invitation to write a special article may come very early in your career or at the point where you have developed national visibility. Early in your career, your mentor may receive such an opportunity and ask you if you are willing to draft (and coauthor) an invited contribution.   This can present a wonderful chance to get another publication, but it will involve considerable time and effort on your part. I would encourage you to say yes, if offered, but be certain that you can deliver. Make sure you understand the specifications and the timeline. Is the deadline flexible or relatively fixed?

As with other invitations, do not take something on unless you can produce. Here is some background information that will help you decide to accept the invitation and ensure that you are able to fulfill your role well. Communicate with your mentor or the person who invited you if circumstances change and you anticipate significant delay. Do not assume that the deadline is flexible or padded.

There are two major scenarios that lead to this invitation: a general invitation to submit, and an invitation to contribute to a special issue. Each is considered individually below. Because many of these manuscripts will take the form of review articles, see Chapter 5 for additional tips.

General Invitation to Submit. Let's say that your mentor is on the editorial board of a journal and has promised the editor-in-chief to contribute a review article on a specific topic. Here, the deadline is relatively flexible, and you may have considerable input into the exact topic or subtopic. This will presumably be an area familiar to you and your mentor. Journals usually solicit review articles as a way of increasing value to readers and of improving the Impact Factor. The editor-in-chief may have identified that articles on bariatric surgery, for example, are heavily cited and downloaded, and that it would be timely to publish a review article on this topic. Your mentor, an expert in the area, has agreed to submit an article. You may, in fact, have amassed a considerable amount of material on a side topic (for example, the use of a particular technique) during the course of writing a research paper, and this may present a perfect opportunity to use that material.

It is important to recognize that your finished paper will be submitted for peer review, critiqued, reviewed, and may be rejected just like any other manuscript. This generic invitation to contribute does not come with any guarantee of acceptance or any offer of special treatment. Sometimes young authors (and even more senior individuals) are surprised or miffed if a solicited manuscript is rejected. Sometimes perfectly good manuscripts are rejected, simply because the editor has accepted another review article on the same topic in the interim. And, of course, by definition peer-reviewed journals follow a peer review process, and that may result in rejection.

If the manuscript is rejected, you then submit it to another journal and, if the topic is indeed timely and the manuscript well-written, it is likely that you will be able to secure publication. The mature thing to do is to recognize that the invitation to submit provided you the impetus to write the paper, regardless of where it is ultimately published.

So, all things considered, an invitation to submit provides a great opportunity and I would urge you to enthusiastically accept (unless you feel unable to complete the project).

Invitation to Contribute to a Special Issue. Things are a bit different if you are dealing with an invitation to submit to a special issue of the journal (for example, an issue devoted to bariatric surgery), a publication such as "Surgical Clinics of North America" or a Festschrift (see below). This invited submission will have a tight deadline and more detailed specifications that may or may not mesh well with your current knowledge and interests. You must carefully honor those specifications and that deadline.

The major benefit of this sort of invitation is that acceptance is much more likely because your paper goes into a special group of manuscripts that are being collated for a specific purpose. In a sense, your manuscript fits into a designated niche and the issue would be diminished without it. The peer review process still occurs, and you may need to respond to reviewers' comments on a very tight timeline, but you are assured that the journal *wants* your manuscript.

Once again, unless you are certain you cannot complete the assignment on time and to specifications, I would urge you to accept. Some specific categories of invited submissions are briefly discussed in the sections that follow.

Invited Review Articles versus State of the Art Papers

An **invited review article** is just that – a review article (see Chapter 5) on a specific topic. Before embarking on this project, do a careful literature search with special reference to the journal which has solicited the review article.

A **state of the art paper** usually summarizes current research or knowledge in a particular field. It often deals with a topic in which there have been recent developments, or where significant unresolved issues remain. It may go on to highlight promising areas for further research. The person asked to provide this manuscript is usually an active investigator in the field. The only difference between this and a review article is the singular focus on the forefront of knowledge on the topic. It may be appropriate for you to refer to prior published works of your own. While including data from those papers may enrich your article, avoid including new unpublished data. Once it is published, even in this format, you should not submit it for publication elsewhere.

Festschrifts

A Festschrift is a collection of papers honoring the career of a living senior luminary person. Typically, papers are solicited from mature trainees or mentees of a particularly influential individual. Usually an introductory page or two details the career of the person who is being honored.

Thus, unless you are the person organizing the Festschrift, your task is to write a paper that brings together various aspects of your own work in the overall context of the state of the art in your area of research. Rarely will you be instructed to refer directly to the honoree or how that person helped shape your career – avoid this unless you are instructed to the contrary.

Your contribution is best envisioned as a "state of the art" paper. It may quite naturally highlight work that you did with the honored individual, or it may diverge into a totally different field of endeavor – in which case the connection may be less obvious to you. You were chosen as an exemplar of the influence that your mentor had over the entire field. Your paper then becomes part of a collection that is published in a specific journal. Usually this will have been arranged ahead of time, so you will know which journal (and thus, which readership) you are writing for. You should expect to receive instructions including deadline, length, format, and so on. Do not hesitate to speak with the person organizing the Festschrift, if you are unsure of your role. Simply typing Festschrift into the search field of PubMed will generate a long list of examples.

A final word: contributing to a Festschrift sometimes causes anxiety way out of proportion to the task at hand. Recognize that this you are no longer a trainee under this powerful individual; you are a fully mature contributor in your own right. Separate the writing task from any memories of your association with the person being honored. Ambivalence is part of most human relationships; recognize it, acknowledge it, and move forward with the task at hand.

Point – Counterpoint

Here your assigned task is to argue in favor of one side in a debate. You will be paired with another expert who will similarly argue for the other side. You will have been chosen because you have published on the side for which you are advocating. Generally, it is thus easy to summarize the body of evidence in favor of your chosen approach. Often the space assigned for this point-counterpoint dialogue is at most the space for one article, your portion occupies half of this space, and thus you must make every word count.

Difficulties may arise if, since writing on this topic, you have shifted your point of view. This is particularly common in surgery, where trends may arise and sweep through the surgical community in a year or so. If this is the case, immediately notify the editor who has solicited your point. The editor is then free to choose another individual. Resist the temptation to write from a point of view that you no longer believe to be valid.

Editorials and Invited Commentaries

Editorials and invited commentaries help put a paper (or sometimes several papers on the same topic published in a single edition) into perspective by summarizing how these papers contribute to knowledge in the field. Excellent examples of these can be found in JAMA, the New England Journal of Medicine, and Science. They are usually solicited from experts not involved in the papers being published.

Letters to the Editor

Letters to the editor provide a way for readers to communicate important information to the editor. Most commonly, they deal with questions raised by (or controversy with) published authors. Several letters may be collated into a group and the authors of the manuscript given an opportunity to respond.

The most important things to remember are: be objective and remain civil. If you are on the receiving end of the critiques, you will inevitably feel a bit stung and maybe even peevish. Set your feelings aside and thank the writers for bringing up these interesting points. Then proceed to address the points, much as you might address reviewers' comments (Chapter 10) but in a manner suitable for publication. Look at back issues of the journal for guidance; failing that, excellent examples are found in JAMA and the New England Journal of Medicine.

Some journals allow the publication of short clinical or research observations as letters to the editor. This may be a way to get some genuinely new material published rapidly when a full manuscript and the accompanying submission process seems inappropriate. This is, in general, a very difficult route to pursue and is not recommended.

Continuing Medical Education (CME) materials

Attendees at CME events are generally given a (paper or electronic) collection of enduring materials to supplement the actual presentations. A variety of formats are utilized, and the CME organization may request a specific format (such as an outline) or may leave the choice up to you. Think about the CME events that you may have attended, and what sort of format you felt was useful.

Here are a couple of possible formats, with tips for maximizing your efficiency and the value to your audience.

- **Narrative format** – Very few CME organizations still request this type of material. Generally the page count is severely limited. Think of this as a very concise review or state of the art paper. Consider leveraging this effort by subsequently expanding it to a full length manuscript of that type (and acknowledging the previous presentation). Unless the CME organization requests a narrative format, generally an outline or annotated slide format is easier for you and better for your audience.

- **Annotated slides** – This is arguably the best format for attendees. Simply take your final slide presentation and pull it into a word processing document. You can then annotate your slides, providing additional narrative material, notes, or references. Leave room for notes. This format is commonly used to produce material to supplement medical student lectures. It works equally well for CME purposes. Do not change your slides after turning in your handout, unless you want to watch (and hear) your audience frantically shuffle papers.

- **Outline** – An outline format can be effective, especially if you include space for folks to insert their own notes.

- **References** – Include selected references, possibly as an annotated list, with any CME materials.

- **Reprints** – It may be possible to include reprints of your own or other authors' work in your packet under the "fair use" copyright provision. Do not assume this to be the case. Notify the CME organization well before the deadline, so that they can address any copyright issues.

Writing Multiple Choice Questions (MCQ's)

Journals typically choose about four articles and offer continuing medical education (CME) or maintenance of certification (MOC) credit. This is an added benefit for subscribers. Typically the reader must answer four questions and is rewarded with one hour of credit.

If you are asked to write MCQ's for these purposes, here are a few tips for producing high value questions.

- Start with the premise that you want to reinforce key learning points from your presentation or manuscript.
- List those key points.
- Devise an MCQ for each key point.
- Write a concise paragraph explaining why one answer is correct and the others are wrong.

MCQ's typically begin with a narrative introduction (called the "stem") and then a series of options. Stick to a simple format, where there is one correct answer and several (typically 3 to 4) incorrect answers, technically termed "distractors." All options should be similar in type and length (that is, if the correct answer is a diagnostic maneuver, *all* of the options should be diagnostic maneuvers).

Avoid the abstruse. While you may be enthralled with the minutiae of your study or the specialized statistical methodology employed in your data analysis, limit yourself to major points.

Similarly, avoid answers of the form "start an IV and obtain a CT scan." These two-part answers are unnecessarily complex and may become tricky, rewarding the good test-taker rather than someone who has honestly learned the material.

Because most journals now include CME or MOC credits as a benefit for subscribers, you can easily find examples. As you work through this material, you will readily see the difference between a good question and a bad one. Emulate the good ones, and learn from (stylistically) the bad ones.

The National Board of Medical Examiners ® (NBME) provides a useful "Item Writing Manual" through its website (http://www.nbme.org/publications/item-writing-manual.html). The section on multiple choice questions with one best answer is most nearly applicable to CME questions. Note that NBME format begins with a clinical stem, whereas CME questions may or may not. The NBME material provides particularly good examples of good and bad questions.

Finally, for each question, supply a paragraph explaining why only one answer is correct and the others are wrong.

Chapter 8. Getting Started
Kent Choi MD

This chapter ties together ideas from the preceding chapters and introduces some new issues, such as authorship, that are best faced early in the writing process.

Authorship

Authorship of research work confers credit and is a formal recognition of the intellectual input of an individual. It also assigns the responsibility of the publication to the individual. All named authors must be willing to accept public responsibility for their part in the publication. Most of the major research institution, publication companies or journals will have published guideline regarding authorship.

There are very few single author papers. Most projects involve several people. How do you decide who is an author? A small group of editors of medical journals met informally in Vancouver, British Columbia in 1978 to establish guidelines for the format of manuscripts submitted to their journals. This effort has expanded to form the International Committee of Medical Journal Editors (ICMJE), which broadened its scope to include guidelines on several key topics, including authorship (http://www.icmje.org/).

The right to authorship is not tied to position or profession and does not depend on whether the contribution was paid for or voluntary. It is not enough to have provided materials or routine technical support, or to have collected that data on which the publication is based. Substantial intellectual involvement is required.

According to the ICMJE, attribution of authorship must be based on substantial contributions (http://www.icmje.org/recommendations/browse/roles-and-responsibilities/defining-the-role-of-authors-and-contributors.html) such as:
- Conception and design of the project, and
- Analysis and interpretation of research data, and
- Drafting significant parts of the work or critically revising it so as to contribute to the interpretation.

One author should take responsibility for the integrity of the work as a whole from inception to published article. This individual is identified as the corresponding author who must agree to be accountable for all aspects of the work, and to ensure that questions related to the accuracy or integrity of any part of the work are appropriately investigated and resolved.

What order do the names go in? There are many different ways to list the co-authors for any particular publication. Typically the first author is the most important individual, and the last author is a senior person who may be the corresponding author. Additional authors are then listed in rough order of their contributions. Variation exists among different disciplines, research groups, institutions, countries, and cultures. In fact, there *are* no particular guidelines for determining the order of authors. In general, simple seniority should not be a consideration in deciding the author order.   The order of authorship should be a joint decision of all the co-authors. When there are multiple authors, settle the issues of authorship up front, in writing if necessary. Every author must have contributed to the paper and must be willing to take responsibility for it.

Types of authors. The first author, or the lead author, should be the primary architect of the entire project. Commonly, he or she is primarily responsible for the study design, publication drafting, and may be the corresponding author (see below). In short, the first author is the one who did the bulk of the intellectual work. However, the lead author does not have to be the principal investigator or project leader. When a student works on a project as his or her thesis, the student should be the lead author.

The last author, or the senior author, is often the senior faculty member who has been instrumental throughout the entire project in advisory role, may have provided funding and laboratory space, and has critically reviewed and edited the manuscript. The last author will sometimes be the corresponding author, especially in the situation when the first author is still in training status. This is a matter of practicality; the trainee will probably move to another institution and may be difficult to reach; the senior author is usually more stable. Because of the active involvement of the last author, this role is fundamentally different from that of an honorary author.

Often the first and last authorship positions are the most coveted.

74

The other co-authors are those listed after the first author and before the last one. The order of this list, in general, implies no special hierarchy, unless specified by the authors. The first author should, however, be sensitive to the feelings of those in the middle of the list, who will sometimes obsess over the order of names.

Some journals have limited the number of author names listed on the table of contents. A good general rule is "not to have more authors than patients" – this is especially cited for case reports! In addition, the U.S. National Library of Medicine (NLM) lists in MEDLINE only the first 24 names plus the last author's when there are more than 25 authors. How do you end up with more than 25 authors? Most such papers are huge multi-institutional studies with principle investigators and support researchers at numerous sites. This is unlikely to be a situation that a neophyte writer will encounter.

Honorary authorship is generally condemned. Senior faculty members sometimes attach their names to work done in their laboratory, department, or division as a matter of course. This may sometimes confuse with the concept of the last author role since the most senior person tend to be listed as last author.

This practice occurs sometimes due to local politics or expectation, sometime as unwritten agreement among researchers to add each other's names to help bolster their CV. It has led to a proliferation in the number of authors listed, sometimes given a veneer of respectability to faulty work, and serves only to pad the CV's of senior faculty. For this reason, many journals require that the role of each author be explicitly stated. In addition, each author will need to sign an attestation statement. This practice helps avoid the reverse situation, where a junior person puts a more senior person on as coauthor without checking with the senior person.

Ghost authors are professional writers (often paid by commercial sponsors) whose role is not acknowledged. They are invisible. Some institutions employ professional writers whose job it is to write manuscripts. This is more common when material is being written for a lay than for a professional audience. More commonly, a professional writer may be employed to help edit manuscripts and get them ready for publication. Such writers rarely meet ICMJE criteria to qualify as authors and hence are not listed. There is a difference between institutionally-employed writers and those paid for by a commercial sponsor. The latter may introduce a potential conflict of interest. Ethically, it is important that you disclose the situation to the audience.

The other contributors include all individuals made direct contribution to the project but did not merit authorship. The author may wish to express their gratitude to these individuals. This can be done under the Acknowledgements section, typically at the end of the publication.

Working with co-authors. Typically, a research idea is generated by few individuals based on a personal thought process or a conversation with colleagues. However, completing the project typically involves a small group with similar interests. It is important to "meet" as a group periodically to exchange ideas and to divide up the work and the responsibility. These meetings can be simple e-mail chains rather than face-to-face meetings, but communication among the group is essential. Generally only one person can write the paper, but the work (obtaining IRB approval, doing the literature search, summarizing the literature, data collection and analysis, and writing up the results) can be divided. Habits that are developed during this type of writing become valuable later when working with co-authors on larger projects such as grants, chapters or books.

While it is ideal for the group to decide up front who will be authors, and even what order the names will appear, it is not unusual for names to be added or dropped, or the order changed as the project progresses. This can happen when someone is unable to carry out his or her assigned task and another person is pulled in, or when it becomes obvious that additional expertise in a particular area is needed. Clear communication, tact, and sensitivity can help avoid hurt feelings.

Avoid embarrassing situations by clearly communicating your intent to publish with your coauthors. Particularly when authors come from more than one department, it is not rare to learn that a coauthor in another department has submitted some or all of your data to a journal in their own discipline. In an extreme case, this may preclude you from publishing your paper, because duplicate publication is considered such a grave offense in medical publishing.

Authorship can get political. As a junior person, you may find yourself in a difficult situation where someone (often your supervisor) insists on being an author, but has not contributed to the work. Or you may find that a proposed coauthor does not deliver what you need. Keep your focus on the project, the needs of the project, and enlist your coauthors and published criteria for authorship if necessary. The book "Publishing and Presenting Clinical Research," referenced at the end of this chapter, includes specific scripts to use for a variety of very thorny political situations.

Maintaining Focus and Balance in your Writing

As you begin writing, maintain focus by remembering your readers and keeping in mind the basic question - what does the reader need to know in order to understand the fundamental message of your paper? Maintain balance by not overloading the paper with unrelated details. As a general rule, you need to be familiar with the material at least one level deeper than you plan to write. Use this deeper level as a foundation but do not incorporate minutiae in your paper.

It is easy to get too deep and off track. A literature search often produces much information that may or may not relate to your fundamental message. It is often counterproductive to jam every reference into the paper. You may be less tempted to put everything in if you keep in mind that nothing needs to be wasted - you can always use this additional material for a book chapter or review article.

The Mechanics of Putting it all Together

Be precise! What is the central hypothesis and what are the aims that the paper/study seeks to answer? For hypothesis-driven research, this is easy. Put your hypothesis up front and close with it at the end (think of bookends). To answer the questions of 1) why do you want to present this paper – background and introduction; 2) how are you going to answer the research question – methods and materials; 3) what do you found out – result and findings; 4) what does the finding mean and why – discussion and conclusion.

Work through the sections, but not necessarily in order. Many writers start with the methods and results sections, and use the momentum generated from this to drive through the discussion and to circle back to the introductory material. The logic is that the methods and results section simply describe what you did and what you found, but the introduction and discussion require putting your results into context. Conclusions must be based on your results or findings. Don't overstate your case. The abstract is often either the first (in the case of material submitted to a meeting) or the last finished product.

How to Research and Organize your Material.
While this book does not specifically deal with the design and execution of research studies, a few words are in order. Time and effort spent before and during data collection and analysis will pay off with better data and an easier job writing up the project. Sloppy work in the beginning may result in an unpublishable manuscript and a huge waste of time and energy.

First generate your research question and identify your central hypothesis. List or outline the aims and objectives. Frequently a junior faculty may be given a task to review a decade or two of surgical experience within the department/institution in managing a specific problem (for example, the surgical management of chronic pancreatitis).

It is tempting to simply collect and analyze the data, without any specific research question, and then see what you have. Most experienced researchers will discourage this approach, which is sometimes called "data dredging". Instead, start with a question based on your knowledge and expertise regarding the topic. You and your mentor may have noticed, for example, that fewer longitudinal pancreatojejunostomies are being done at your institution. Is this a trend? Are more resections being performed? How have advanced interventional radiology and endoscopy changed surgical practice? Formulate your hypothesis. It could be a simple one, such as "stenting is being used more and surgical ductal decompression is being used less."

Always obtain Institutional Review Board approval *before* beginning data collection.

It is certainly possible that your data may not be sufficient to address the research question you have, but that another result of interest is obtained. It is perfectly fine to redirect your research to answer a slightly different question, or to follow clues that emerge as you analyze your data. This approach will allow you to explore and discuss the original question to the extent your data allows.

Once the research question and central hypothesis are established, the aims and objective of the research activity can be developed the using an outline, a fishbone diagram or even a concept map. An outline is still the best way to organize your information, as it will flow naturally into the linear structure of the discussion section of the paper. There will frequently be some cross-reference from one section to another. Thus, the paragraph on pathogenesis may share similar concepts with treatment strategies, because pathogenesis dictates treatment.
This will be revisited when you write the discussion section of your paper. Establish a time schedule so that each task will have a due date.

Reviewing and citing the literature, and avoiding plagiarism which is an increasing concern among publishers. It is something you, as an author, want to avoid at all costs. It is defined as an act or instance of using or closely imitating the language and thoughts of another author without authorization and the representation of that author's work as one's own, as by not crediting the original author. It can be deliberate or inadvertent. Inadvertent plagiarism sometimes occurs when material is accumulated during a literature search and stored in a sloppy fashion. Here are some tips to help stay organized and avoid this pitfall.

The mechanics of a literature search is rather simple. The key is to keep all of the data organized. Setting up folders of references or index card system (either paper or electronic) will save much time later and it will allow you to be able to retrieve the information for future projects. Remember that your ultimate goal as a writer is to develop an area of expertise; having written once on a topic you are likely to revisit it in the future. For each reference folder, include a brief summary of the literature and anticipated usage in the project, background material or quotation in discussion; list key points of articles either with bullets or quotations.

To avoid inadvertent plagiarism, copy any quotes word for word into your notes and place these in quotation marks. You may then rephrase these or keep as direct quotes as seems appropriate (in either case, you will cite the source).
Be especially careful if using notes from which you have lectured. Sometimes experienced authors accumulate files of their own lecture notes from which they eventually produce a textbook.

These files of notes, not originally intended for publication, often lack attribution, and inadvertent plagiarism results. Avoid this by developing sound scholarly habits from the beginning of your career.

Keep in mind the distinction between "Fair use" and the Copyright law (http://www.copyright.com/Services/copyrightoncampus/basics/fairuse.html). Information in the public domain, such as newspaper stories, journal articles, and information on public webpages, can be cited with proper referencing. This is commonly considered fair use of public knowledge. Scholarly works generally demand citation of sources, even if copyright law does not.

Art works or graphic, photograph, and slide shows or movie clips are generally considered to be copyright protected materials. Proper permission (and often a sizeable fee) is required to use these materials in your publication. If you simply want to include an illustration from *your own* previous publication, most publishers will waive the fee. You still need to obtain permission.

The Literature Search

Do three literature searches, at least. You will have done a thorough literature search before embarking upon the project. As you start to write the paper, do another literature search to find out what is new in the field. When you are ready to put the paper in the mail, do a third literature search to identify any fresh material that should be cited or addressed in your discussion.

Learn how to use reference management software, so that you can import references directly into a database that you subsequently use in your manuscript and future work on the topic.

How to Organize the Material

Identify logical subheadings, either through an outline or a fishbone diagram or concept map. Use these as pages in a notebook or put them on cards. Cards are particularly useful, because you can group them in various combinations and move them around. Accumulate information under each subheading. Throughout the process of drafting the manuscript, it is very important to maintaining focus on the key messages that you wish to deliver. Each point should be generated by your data and connected to information obtained from your review of the

80

literature. Your scholarly craftsmanship will be demonstrated in your own synthesis of the materials.

Safeguarding your Data

Obviously, any research involving patients (including retrospective chart reviews) will require IRB approval and part of that approval process will involve describing how you will safeguard the data. Beyond that, keeping your original data safe is absolutely critical. Whether it is in a secure reference folder, or as the original raw data (again, in a secure folder), all the analysis results are crucial not only to verify the validity of the research outcome but also to help address reviewer comments and questions, as well as rebut any unfounded criticisms.

Presenting Data with Tables versus Graphs versus Narrative Within the Text

Most journals have limitations and guidelines about how many tables or graphs you may put into your manuscript. Consider your audience and the style of the publication you are aiming at. See Chapter 6 for a discussion of various data presentation formats. What is appropriate for a general medical journal may not be appropriate for a specialty publication.
The key is to provide the reader with the clearest and best picture of your data.

If you are simply comparing two groups on a few categories, it may be possible to imbed some of your data in the text. When there are several groups, or interaction between variables may be significant, a table or graph may be better. Avoid duplication. Do not cite specific numeric data in the text if it is given in a table or graph or table.

Do not draw conclusions in the results section – thus, avoid statements such as "nearly twice as many infections occurred in Group I as in Group II (Table 1)". Use a simple phrase such as "The rate of infection in the two groups is given in Table 1." The general rule here is economy of words. Here you simply give the data and the analysis results. In your discussion, you can restate and summarize and give conclusions.

In general, putting all of your results in your text is detailed but cumbersome; a graph can present a series of data and deliver a single message (for example, time trends) in a manner that is easy to perceive; a table can present a large amount of data in an organized fashion and deliver more than one message. This is discussed in greater detail in Chapter 6, Reports of Original Research.

Graphs and other Visual Aids

Keep these simple, clear, and visually honest. There are many types of graphs. Histograms or bar graphs are used to compare things between different groups or to track changes over time. Line graphs are used to track changes over periods of time. Pie charts are useful when you are discussing relative parts of a whole. X-Y plots, including scatter plots, are used to illustrate the relationship between the two different variables and show, in a very visual way, the dispersal of individual data points around the regression line. Area graphs are combination of line graphs and X-Y plots. They can be used to track changes over time for one or more groups in more than one dimension. Always use the simplest and clearest way of displaying your data.

Illustrations

The decision on using photographs versus line drawings are best addressed by asking which one achieves the best demonstrates your ideas. Photographs are essential for pathologic findings, skin lesions, and radiographs. Take care that the photograph is high quality and does not include extraneous detail or patient identifiers. Modern electronic publishing and decreased cost of color reproduction have made it rare to encounter a journal that limits use of color.

If you are trying to illustrate steps in a technical procedure, you can use either photographs or line drawings. You may want to consider having both (for example, to show a key finding during surgery) - a photograph to show the actual finding, and an accompanying line drawing as a kind of key. Always consider the journal requirements and typical style, and the potential financial impact of your choice. Photographs are generally free of cost to you, but more apt to include details that are not of interest to your readers.

Line drawings may convey the essence of a procedure better, but can be costly to have drawn. It may be tempting to draw your own; if so, have a colleague objectively assess the quality of the final product. Even if your final drawing is not "publication quality" it can serve as a template for a professional medical illustrator.

Working with a Medical Illustrator

This is a consultant service. The quality of the product depends on who is the medical illustrator but the quality control is up to you. There are some helpful reference guidelines available on-line by the Association of Medical Illustrators, including an excellent "Client Guideline" (http://ami.org/).

What artwork do you need? Use whatever you need to demonstrate your main message. It should be just enough to make it clear. Keep the audience and their needs in mind. A simple line drawing can emphasize key points and eliminate extraneous information. Medical illustrators are expert at creating art as a communication tool for medical professionals.

A skilled medical illustrator can work from a photograph, a video clip, or a rough sketch. An illustrator who can produce art rapidly and to your specifications is invaluable; many productive authors find and cultivate an ongoing relationship with a particular artist. When working with an artist, it is very important to make certain that the others understand the key points to be conveyed. One should supply supporting material or documentation, such as photographs, drawings, or other illustrations, to help the artist to understand what is important.

Anticipate significant cost for custom art. A single plate may cost several hundred dollars. If you are a skilled artist, you may try to do the work yourself. You may want to consult with a medical illustrator for guidance. There are certain conventions. Make sure you observe them. There are certain regulations with regarding styles, line width, and size (typically drawings are made larger than publication size, with thicker lines, to allow for reduction. The reduction also helps "hide" any minor imperfections in the line).

Digital art has gradually hand drawing but still requires time and thought. The fundamental question remains the same – do you need to artwork to display your message or does to act out more delivery your main message better?

You may be able to reprint art works with permission from other authors and the publisher. You may have to pay a fee, which can easily be around $1000. You are less likely to have to pay a fee if you know the editor who grants permission and if you make a case that this will, by enhancing your visibility, help rather than hurt the earlier publication.   Even if you can borrow the art for free, you will need a high quality original (or digital original) to submit for publication, and this can be problematic.

When considering color versus black and white art works, quality of reproduction is crucial. Does the added color provide additional information? As noted above, most journals allow color illustrations, but a few will require you to provide funds to cover this.

Drafts and Revisions

The first draft is just to get it down on paper. The second draft is to get it organized. Many experienced authors advocate writing long (that is, lots of words) for the first draft, then cutting significantly with each successive draft. Several more drafts are often needed to polish the final product.

You must do a final literature search just before sending it in. Typically several months will have passed, and you do not want to ignore new publications (possibly from authors who will be asked to review your own manuscript). This not only improves your paper but may also allow you to avoid unnecessary criticism from reviewers.

As you draft the manuscript, maintain focus on the key messages that you wish to deliver. Each major point should develop naturally from your data and be put into the context of previous literature. Your craftsmanship is demonstrated from your own synthesis of the materials.

The number of references should reflect the nature of the topic and the type of paper and journal. An established but controversial topic will always have more references than a truly novel idea or new trial. Review articles tend to cite more references than case reports, to give two extremes. Chapters vary, depending upon the style of the book. Inadequate referencing may be criticized by the reviewers as a sign of an inadequate exploration of the topic. Conversely, listing too many references rarely results in rejection of your paper; at worst, you may be asked to trim the list.

Use reference management software to simplify the tedious task of formatting and changing the order of references.

Good software will also allow you to formulate a comprehensive reference list that you can dip into for subsequent papers on the same or related topics.

The "Journal Log"
Keep track of submissions. Establish a subfolder in your computer, or keep a paper journal (a spiral bound notebook will suffice) where you can list the crucial information for each manuscript. Thus, in a spiral bound notebook, use a new page for each manuscript. Write down the crucial dates - submitted, returned with critique, resubmitted, accepted, galleys, publication. This will allow you to go through this periodically and look for material that may not have ever been published. Periodically take one of these out, update it, send it out, and you may be pleasantly surprised. It is a good habit to develop and log a fallback strategy - where to submit next if you are rejected by your first choice (for further details, see Chapter 14).

Chapter 9. Submitting Your Manuscript
Scott Sherman MD

Edit, edit, and re-edit your manuscript before you submit it. Let
trusted and experienced colleagues read it. If you are fortunate
enough to know someone who is willing to go over it in detail with
you, by all means take them up on it. It will take multiple drafts to
get your manuscript into shape for submission for publication. This
is time well spent.

Generally, as you revise, continue to tighten and condense.
Beginning writers are often afraid that they just won't have enough
material. The journal editor, on the other hand, is concerned with
page count and wants to publish as much top-quality material
without exceeding the journal budget. Although this is less of a
problem with electronic publishing, many highly prestigious
journals consider the electronic version as an alternative to the
print version. Strive to be concise but complete.

Whereas previous chapters dealt with specific forms of
papers, this chapter deals with the actual submission process. This
is the final common pathway for any form of writing that is to be
published in a medical journal.

How to Submit Your Manuscript
The decision to submit always involves a compromise
between wanting to include just a little more, and wanting to have
the project finished. Nevertheless, at some point after many rounds
of editing, your manuscript will meet all formatting and length
requirements, will have been extensively proofread, and will have
all figures and tables perfectly arranged. You are ready to send it to
your target journal.

While online submission websites have streamlined the
process considerably, it is best to allow several hours for this
process and expect difficulties with the website. When confronting
a deadline, do not leave submission to the last minute. Begin the
process by creating a user account and log in several days prior to
when you plan to finalize the submission. Some journals require all
authors to fill out conflict of interest forms prior to submission,
and this is not always obvious from the author instructions.
Investigating the website in advance therefore helps avoid last-
minute scrambling. Once you have uploaded all documents,

figures, and required forms, a .pdf version of your manuscript will be compiled.

Carefully proofread this and make sure it looks the way you want it to, as this will be the version that reviewers will receive. At this point you will discover the one small typo you missed despite all your prior efforts, and it is worth the time to correct it, re-upload your document, re-review the new pdf, and repeat this process until your submission is perfect.

Submit Your Manuscript to Just One Journal at a Time

Generally, as part of the submission process, you will have to attest that this is the only place to which you are sending your manuscript. The ICMJE statement on duplicate publication (http://www.icmje.org/recommendations/browse/ publishing-and-editorial-issues/overlapping-publications.html) clearly explains the rationale behind this policy. Acceptable instances of overlapping publication are discussed in that policy (see also Chapter 2). You will, of course, have compiled a list of potential journals – avoid the temptation to send your manuscript to more than one of them!

Before Finalizing your Submission

When you are ready to submit, perform one last literature search in case new publications have appeared. Make sure you have included these and addressed them in your discussion.

Do this for two reasons: first, it is the scholarly correct thing to do. Second, it is quite possible that the editor-in-chief will go to PubMed to find a reviewer who has published recently in your field, so you may find yourself in the rather awkward position of being reviewed by an author whose recent work you did not acknowledge.

Read the beginning and end of your paper and ask yourself these questions, which will be addressed in the material which follows:

- Did I make the case for doing this scholarly work (and indirectly, for publication)?
- Did I carefully explain the similarities and differences between my results and those of others?
- Does the end of the paper wrap it all up?
- Does the title accurately reflect what the manuscript says?

- Have I overstated my conclusions, or is every point that I make supported by my data?
- Have I chosen my keywords well?

Did I make the case for my work? The case is usually first stated briefly in the abstract and expanded slightly in the introductory paragraph. Research may carve new paths, may be confirmatory, or may provide additional data in a field where existing data diverge. Which category best describes your material? If your study is confirmatory, you will need to take especial pains to explain why another paper should be published in this particular field.

In the case of a review article, why did you choose to delve into this particular question at this time? Maybe there is new information that you want to highlight for your fellow clinicians. Maybe nothing has been published in the past decade. Make the editor and reviewers, your first readers, care about the contents of your manuscript.

Did I carefully explain the similarities and differences between my results and those of others? This is the role of the Discussion section. With your updated literature search in hand, go methodically through all of the various aspects of your topic that you want to highlight. If your results are confirmatory, acknowledge this. If your results diverge from those of others, or if studies in the literature differ in their conclusions, then carefully describe the similarities and differences.

Do not hypothesize or overstate your conclusions (see below)! Also use this section to frankly acknowledge any limitations of your study. Double-check to make sure that this section doesn't simply repeat the Results section. Remember that the Results section should summarize your data; the Discussion should put it into perspective.

With your latest literature search in hand, ideally one performed minutes before your final edit, modify your discussion to incorporate any significant new studies.

Does the end of the paper wrap it all up? The last paragraph should summarize your conclusions. Some journals use a format with an actual "Summary" or "Conclusions" section, but many will leave it up to you. If the journal does not have a designated section for your wrap up, the final paragraph might begin "In summary, we found…" or "In conclusion, we found…" to alert the reader that this is where you pull it all together.

Unfortunately, most of your readers will simply glance at the abstract; those that actually read the paper will concentrate on the introduction and the conclusions.

Does the title accurately reflect what the manuscript says? Again, make sure that your title is concise, accurate, and does not overstate your results. Scan several issues of the journal and get a sense of the general style used for titles. Remember, the title is the thing that will get readers interested in your paper. Make every word count.

Have I overstated my conclusions, or is every point that I make supported by my data? Identify your conclusions and backtrack through the manuscript to confirm a tight chain of data and logical reasoning. Often additional work remains to be done – acknowledge this with a simple statement such as "While these data support the hypothesis that _____, randomized prospective clinical trials remain to be done."

Have I chosen my keywords well? You only have a limited number of keywords. Use them well. Don't hesitate to consult a medical librarian if in doubt.

Suggested Reviewers

Some journals will require you to submit the names of suggested reviewers. These people must be outside of your own institution, and it is therefore possible that you will not know anyone suitable. Your research mentor may be able to suggest qualified (and hopefully sympathetic) colleagues to list. Failing that, you may choose to list senior authors from related publications you have discovered in your literature search. The journal editor may (or may not) pull from your list when sending the manuscript out for review.

The Cover Letter

Your cover letter should be brief and dignified. In most cases, it will simply state that you and your coauthors wish to submit this manuscript for consideration for publication. If you are submitting for a particular feature, for example, "Technical Tips," this is the place to state that.

Use the cover letter to clearly declare any previous publication. If, for example, your work was previously published in another journal in a foreign language and you wish to bring it to an

English-speaking readership, say so. Similarly, if your work is a logical extension of a previously-published study, state this. In both cases, cite the previous publication in the manuscript. In the case of an expanded data set, address this in the text of the manuscript. If possible, append a copy of the previous publication.

Similarly, it never hurts to address up front any declared conflict of interest issues in the cover letter. If you have received funding from a drug company, for example, clarify what sort of funding (e.g. unrestricted research grant, paid speakership).

Chapter 10. Responding to Reviewers' Critiques

Very few manuscripts are accepted "as is." Many writers are given the opportunity to "revise and resubmit." If you are fortunate and have done your job well, you may receive a letter from the editor-in-chief which sounds like a rejection, but which is actually an invitation to revise the manuscript and send it back. Inexperienced authors sometimes read this letter as a true rejection and simply give up.

Here is what to do. Do it in a timely, humble, and sincere fashion. Follow these steps and your revised manuscript *may* be accepted by the journal. Even if it is rejected on resubmission, you will almost surely have improved the manuscript and you can then submit it (in the new, improved form) to another journal.

If you have never served as an invited reviewer for a journal, read Chapter 12 as well as this chapter. The more that you understand the review process, the better you will be able to respond to critiques.

When is a Rejection Letter not a Rejection?

When you send off a paper (or a proposal for that matter) and get back an email or electronically formatted letter that reads something like this "the editors are interested in your paper provided you address the following critiques" by all means do so. Even if the phraseology is more lukewarm, you should immediately start revising.

The editors may express a high level of interest or a low level of interest. It is not unusual for novice writers to mistake a low level of interest for a flat-out rejection when, in fact, the editors are willing to consider a major revision. If you are uncertain, ask a more experienced colleague to read the letter and give you an unbiased assessment.

What you need to do. You will need to answer each critique, generating a revised manuscript and a cover letter listing your changes, and get it back to the journal within the specified time frame. The letter from the editor will specify a mechanism for sending your revision back, as well as tell you the format in which the journal wants to receive it. If no deadline is specified by the journal, endeavor to send back your response in a week or two. The longer you delay, the less likely you will complete the task. In addition, the journal may lose interest or the topic may no longer be topical (because someone else has published something similar). Here is a brief checklist:

- Determine the deadline for response
- Go through the list of critiques and separate difficult from easy ones
- Address each critique in the manuscript using "Track changes"
- Compile a cover letter with a complete list of critiques and where and how you addressed them
- Resubmit promptly!

Addressing Critiques

Typically the letter will include two or more lists of critiques from two or more reviewers. The list of critiques may seem daunting indeed – often it extends to two pages. Go down the list and identify the easy points to fix - deal with these first. Keep a list of changes - these will be listed in the cover letter with the revised manuscript.

A simple way to do this is to print out the letter. Check off the easy problems, and encircle the difficult ones. An example of an easy critique might be failure to cite a particular relevant paper. That's easy to fix – look up the paper, cite it and deal with it in your discussion, revise the discussion and renumber the references. Another example of an easy critique might be the common comment, "conclusions are not supported by the data." When you read your manuscript carefully, you may be able to identify the source of the criticism. It is easy to wax eloquent in your concluding enthusiasm. All you really need to do is moderate your language. Other easy matters to fix include the overall length of the paper, grammatical errors, problems with illustrations or tables, and the common confusion between results and discussion (see Chapter 8).

An example of a difficult critique might be a query about data analysis or methodology. If your statistical analysis is challenged, you may need a new statistical consultant. That may even result in a new analysis of your data. If, on the other hand, you planned your experiment and analyzed your data with the assistance of an expert biostatistician, you may simply need to explain your methodology better and document that a biostatistician was involved (both in the manuscript and in your cover letter).

Occasionally a reviewer will wish you had done a different study altogether. For example, a reviewer may recommend that a randomized controlled clinical trial should have been done in place of your retrospective review. Paradoxically, this seemingly fatal flaw is easy to address. The study is the study, the data are the data. Have confidence that the editor would not have invited you to resubmit if they weren't satisfied with your basic methodology. Usually the only way to address this is to acknowledge, in the paper, the need for a follow up randomized clinical trial. Remember, preliminary data (which may be what your paper represents) is the first step toward designing a randomized clinical trial. If your paper is just the last in a long series of retrospective studies that all, essentially, show the same thing, then it really is time for that randomized clinical trial and maybe you should propose one.

When reviewers disagree. It's not unusual for reviewers to disagree. Reviewer A likes a particular aspect of your paper, but reviewer B doesn't. Consider a revision that addresses the problems raised by reviewer B without losing the virtues noted by reviewer A. Adopt that which makes sense and point out in your cover letter what you have done and why. Explain to the editor why you followed one reviewer and not the other. If possible, address the second critique in the manuscript as it may be a point that occurs to readers. At the very least, this may be a point that *confuses* readers, so that a revision for clarity is in order.

When you disagree with a reviewer. Sometimes a reviewer will suggest that a different technique or methodology should have been used. That particular technique may not have been accessible to you when you began the study several years ago. Simply explain the fact, and consider addressing this in the discussion section of the manuscript, perhaps toward the end of the section.

In other cases, the suggested technique or methodology may not be appropriate. In fact, you may be more knowledgeable than the reviewer. This is rare, but it occasionally happens. In this case, you need to convince the editor (and any potential reader) that you are correct. You may need to provide the editor with additional data, copies of relevant papers, etc.

Finally, it is possible that the manuscript is simply not clearly written. Always remember, if the point confused the reviewer and led to an incorrect assessment, it may also confuse the reader. Reword the section for clarity, if possible discussing the potential point of confusion in the manuscript, and explain this to the editor.

Cover Letter

The introductory and concluding text of the cover letter accompanying the revision should be short, succinct, and humble. Begin the cover letter by thanking the editor and reviewers for their time and interest. A single sentence will suffice. Tell the editor you feel that the manuscript is substantially improved (it probably is!)

Then list the critiques, numbering them by reviewer exactly as they were listed in the letter you received from the editor. After each critique, give a short paragraph telling how you addressed the issue. If a particular critique seemed off the mark or two reviewers disagreed, it is fine to mention this in the cover letter but it is still a good idea to make some sort of revision for clarification. If two experienced reviewers were confused, you can bet that the readers will be. Conclude with a statement of gratitude for the opportunity to improve the manuscript.

The Manuscript

In the manuscript itself, use "track changes" to show what you have changed. Each critique, even the ones that seem baseless, should result *in some sort of change* in the manuscript. Sometimes, as noted above, all that is needed is a revision for greater clarity. Authors sometimes explain an issue in the cover letter but fail to make a change in the manuscript. This is a mistake, as it can aggravate an editor taxed with making a final decision. It is always possible to make something clearer and easier to read. Take that critique as an opportunity to do so.

What happens next?

If the criticisms of your manuscript were relatively minor, the editor may make a decision based upon your cover letter and your revised manuscript. If, on the other hand, the critiques were major, the editor may request the same reviewers to read the revised manuscript or may, in some circumstances, ask new reviewers. In any event, you need to make it easy for whoever reads the cover letter and manuscript to see that you have thoroughly and adequately addressed all of the reviewers' concerns.

Dealing with Rejection

Simply addressing all of the reviewers' critiques and sending a nicely revised manuscript and sincere cover letter back to the editor does not guarantee acceptance. Even if you answer all the reviewers' critiques, the paper may be rejected. Sometimes this happens because the editor was just lukewarm about the paper, or a different editor may be assigned to review the revision, or the journal may already have several papers on the topic in the queue and is looking for variety. So the rejection may not have anything to do with the quality of your revised manuscript.

Or, you may have received a clear cut letter of rejection accompanied by critiques. In either case, you should update the literature review, address all the critiques, and send the now-improved manuscript to the next journal on your list (see Chapter 11).

Chapter 11. Dealing with Rejection

Neelima Katragunta MD

After you have worked for months on a manuscript, it is almost impossible not to feel hurt when you receive a rejection letter. Here is a fact that you might want to consider. Prestigious journals reject most of the manuscripts submitted to them. Does that mean all the papers that they reject are "bad" papers? Not necessarily.

Why do journals reject good papers?

The most prestigious journals are inundated with manuscript submissions. Acceptance rates of 5-10% are not rare. The editors sift through numerous manuscripts to find those that will be interesting and useful to their target audience. Sometimes they have to reject good papers for various reasons that may have nothing to do with the quality of the paper.

Understanding these reasons can help you publish your rejected manuscript in another journal, and possibly make your future submissions more likely to be accepted. Some flaws in a manuscript are easy to address while others are not.

Common Problems that can be Fixed

Wrong journal. If you are a novice writer (which you probably are since you are reading this book), you probably have yet to develop the sense for the kind of manuscript that is most likely to be published in a particular journal. A review article on new surgical techniques that has been rejected by multiple surgical journals might, with appropriate modifications, be readily accepted by a primary care journal.

There is a certain hierarchy of journals in any given field. The most prestigious journal in a field might be a lot more stringent and selective than a less prestigious journal. As a new writer, it is best to get some early publications in smaller journals. It will give you both motivation and experience that prepares you to aim for a more prestigious journal down the road. There is nothing wrong with aiming high early on, but submitting to a more appropriate journal might save you a considerable amount of time and possibly some heartache.

Poorly written paper. Poor writing style can easily undermine good science and sound logic. Numerous books (in addition to this brief guide) provide detailed suggestions on how to write well. See Chapter 15 for some selected resources that may help. Remember this: no one is "born" a writer. While some medical writers have both training and the natural ability to write well, most of us can considerably improve their writing style with some help and experience.

Make a compelling case for your paper in the beginning and again at the end. Be clear and concise with your sentences. Make sure there is segue between paragraphs. Use figures and flow charts to elucidate your points. Avoid cluttering your paper with too many abbreviations and obscure terms. Above all be considerate of your reader. Remember that most readers of medical articles have neither the time nor the energy to plough through tedious prose.

English as a second language. A paper is likely to be rejected if the English is poor, even if it is scientifically sound. This problem is, however, easy to address. Seek the help of someone who is both proficient in English and understands the scientific content of your paper. It can be a friend or a colleague that is willing to invest the time and the effort. Remember to pay them back in some thoughtful way. The other option is to hire someone who can do it for you. Some journals offer a low-cost service for aspiring authors who plan to submit to their journal. Consider taking advantage of this.

Topic that is not of interest to journal readership. You may have an elegantly presented paper backed by good science, but it fails to be of any interest to the target audience of a particular journal. See if there is a different journal where this topic might be more relevant, and submit it.

Common Problems that are Difficult to Fix

Bad science. This one is probably a fatal problem for your project. There is not much you can do to salvage it. Use this as an experience to be more careful in designing your future studies. Consider using your literature search to generate a review article, and move on, sadder but wiser.

Overstated results. Sometimes there is nothing really wrong with the study but it just did not produce anything exciting. For example, purely confirmatory or negative results are hard to get published. Again, consider producing a review article using your research.

Your manuscript has been rejected. Now what?

Do *not* pick up the phone or fire off a flaming e-mail to complain loudly to the editors about how unfair you think the decision is, how ignorant the reviewers' comments are, and how terrific you think your paper is. None of the above will help you in getting your manuscript published. Get through your grief response as quickly as possible and move on to the next step. Once you lose momentum, it becomes significantly harder to resurrect a rejected manuscript.

First go through the rejection letter and make sure that you have received a "real" rejection letter, rather than a request to revise and resubmit (see Chapter 10). Generally the letter will make this clear. Ask a senior colleague to read the letter if you are not sure. Get over your initial shock, and read the entire letter through to the end. Seek to understand the reasons for rejection. The critiques that accompany the rejection letter generally allude to them.

Carefully study the reviewers' comments and seek to address them in the revised manuscript. This is important whether or not you will resubmit. Although it is not guaranteed that the new reviewers of your re-submitted manuscript will share the same concerns, it will most probably help improve the appeal of your paper.

You can seek additional information for the reasons of your rejection by sending the editors a short, humble, and extremely polite letter requesting additional feedback. If they do not respond, simply move on.

Once you have identified the reasons for rejection, set about addressing them for your revised manuscript. You can expect to do a considerable amount of rewriting prior to submitting to another journal. Treat it like an entirely new manuscript and go through it thoroughly several times prior to submission.

When to fold? After three or four rejections it may become clear that you have reached the point of diminishing returns. Critiques are contradictory, or none of the letters express any regret or enthusiasm. You may even have tried rewriting the paper for a different audience without success. Sometimes the best thing to do is simply move on to a new project. Do not discard your old material. Set the material aside in a file (either paper or electronic), and continue to add to the file if new material appears in the literature, or if you accumulate additional clinical or experimental data.

Revisiting past failures. Periodically go through your old files and consider your failures - those papers that never got published. Pull out this old material and see if you can send use it somewhere. This is a great thing to do when you are blocked on a major project. The flush of success that you experience from resurrecting an old project and sending it off may translate into momentum that gets you back on track with your current bête noire.

Other uses for the material might surface. A case report can be used as an illustration in a book chapter, for instance. Your research of the topic can be used to generate a review article. If all else fails, publication of some of this material on your website may bring a sense of closure to a project in which you have invested significant time and energy.

Chapter 12. Serving as a Reviewer

As your career unfolds and you publish and present more material, you will inevitably be asked to occasionally review a manuscript for a journal. Typically, the journal will send you an e-mail introducing itself and giving the title (and sometimes the abstract) of the article, along with a deadline and the option to respond yes or no. A typical deadline would be two weeks. How should you proceed?

Why say yes? There are several excellent reasons to say yes. First of all, this involves you in the greater process of peer review, the mechanism by which the scientific literature adds new information. It is part of the citizenship of scholarly activity.

Second, the insights you gain from critically reviewing a manuscript written by another author (and then comparing your review with those of the other two reviewers and the ultimate editor's decision) will help you recognize and correct flaws in your own writing. It helps you be a better writer. You can list "ad hoc reviewer for..." on your curriculum vitae. In time, you may even be invited to join the editorial board.   Finally, journals often offer additional incentives, such as a months' worth of free search engine access, or CME credits for your time.

Why say no? Do not accept an assignment lightly. Give careful consideration to the request. Only agree to review a manuscript if you feel you can do a really good job. A careful review may require 4-6 hours of your time, particularly when you are new at the business. If you are unable to comply with the deadline, refuse the assignment.

If you lack expertise in the topic of the manuscript, refuse. Provide the editors with an alternative reviewer (maybe another faculty member at your institution), if you can. If you are temporarily overloaded with work but would like to be considered in the future, let the journal know that you are unavailable until after a certain date.

Finally, consider your own position – if you have a real or perceived conflict of interest, you must refuse the review.

A polite negative reply might go something like this, "Unfortunately, I must decline this opportunity because _____. You might consider Dr _____ (e-mail _____) as an alternative. I hope you will consider me again in the future," covers most of these and leaves the door open for a future relationship with the journal.

What constitutes a conflict of interest? Common conflicts include: area of scholarship too close to (and hence "competing with") your own, work by a friend or relative, work by a previous trainee, and financial conflicts. Some journals will send you an anonymized manuscript, with authors and institutions removed; others will send you this information only after you accept or decline.

See the section below on "Changing your mind" if you find you need to decline after accepting. If you are uncertain, correspond with the editor of the journal. As in all conflict of interest situations, full disclosure is the rule. After consideration, the editor may decide that your declared conflict is acceptable.

How do journals pick reviewers? First of all, not all submitted manuscripts get reviewed. At some journals, generally the more selective ones, an editor will perform an initial review and reject any manuscript that appears hopeless. While this may appear heartless, it allows the author to submit it to a less selective journal rather than waiting several months to hear back from a journal that was never a realistic choice.

Editors pick their reviewers from the editorial board members, from a list of trusted reviewers in selected topics, and from looking at the bibliography of the submitted manuscript. If you are one of the few people who have published about an obscure condition or complication, you may be asked to review another manuscript on the subject.

Reviewers are added to a database maintained by the journal tracking software. Data available to the editor about you, the reviewer, includes your areas of expertise (often self-identified from a checklist), your response rate (how often you decline a review), how long it takes you to complete a review, your acceptance rate (and how it compares with others). The initial selection of reviewers from this database is typically done by area of expertise. The editor then makes the individual selection after looking at your statistics. The editor is typically most interested in your response rate and how long it takes you to complete a review.

Most journals will try to avoid using any particular reviewer too frequently; however, it is inevitable that reviewers who perform well will be selected preferentially over reviewers who perform badly.

Can you change your mind? Sometimes after accepting a manuscript for review, you find yourself unable or unwilling to complete the task. This may happen because of sudden unexpected time pressures, unanticipated conflicts of interest (most commonly revealed when you see who the authors and institutions are), or because you find yourself deep into science that you do not understand (perhaps because the title doesn't accurately reflect the contents).

Immediately notify the editor and apologize. Go back to the invitation e-mail and reply with a short message explaining the situation and, if possible, suggesting an alternate reviewer. Typically this reply will go to an editorial assistant or managing editor (rather than the editor-in-chief) who will be grateful to you for your frankness. Even after many years as a reviewer, editorial board member, and editor-in-chief, I sometimes find myself in this situation.

This is one reason that I recommend you begin your review process by first glancing at the manuscript – even if you know you will not sit down to read it and review it for a few days.

Will the authors know who I am? At the time of this writing, the vast majority of reviews are still done anonymously. The authors are not told who the reviewers are, nor do reviewers know who the other reviewers are. Only the editor-in-chief knows.

Some reviewers (a very limited number) feel that this is wrong. Those reviewers sign their "Comments for Authors" within the text block. Most journals do not encourage this, and most reviewers feel that this step introduces potential for an unwanted attempt at dialogue. Quite simply, any dialogue between the author and journal should go through the editorial office, not directly from author to reviewer.

This is an area that may change. The journal should make it clear to you what their policy is. In any event, never write something that you cannot stand behind – this is always a good general rule.

What is involved in reviewing a manuscript for a journal?
When you agree to review the manuscript, you will be
directed to a website from which you can read or download the
manuscript, and generally given access to a search engine which
you can use to search for related papers, or search for other
publications by the same authors. Of course, as an academic
author, you will generally have this kind of access through your
institutional library, but using the journal website can be easier
because they "preload" the search fields for you.

You will also have access to a computerized review form.
On the journal website you will also typically find information
about the aims and scope of the journal, and you may find a link to
"Reviewer Guidelines." Follow this link and you will find detailed
information on the review process and various thorny issues,
including ethical violations. I encourage you to take advantage of
these guidelines when you are new at the business of reviewing
papers.

In addition to material supplied by the journal, nationally
accepted guidelines are available on the Internet. COPE (The
Committee on Publication Ethics) guidelines for peer review
contain a checklist that neophyte peer reviewers may find helpful
(http://publicationethics.org/files/Ethical_guidelines_for_peer_re
viewers_0.pdf). Their website contains a wealth of guidelines that
represent the best practices and recommendations of the
international medical publishing community.

A highly comprehensive reference is available online from
the Association of American Medical Colleges (AAMC)
downloadable as a free .pdf (see references at the end).

After your review and (generally) at least one other review
have been received, the editor makes a decision. Many journals give
you access to the (anonymous) comments made by other reviewers
and the final decision letter. This provides an excellent reality check
for your own comments and thoughts. Review these carefully; it
will not only help you become a better reviewer, it will also
ultimately help you as an author.

How do you perform the review? I suggest that until you
are familiar with the process, that you divide the task into three
phases: 1) information gathering, 2) assessment, 3) review. These
phases can unfold sequentially over several days. I recommend that
when you do your first reviews, you take several days to complete

your review so that you have time for reflection. Most of the work of the review can be done offline.

What does a review form look like? Look at the review form for the particular journal. Most contain standard elements. You will be asked if you have any conflicts of interest. Generally, if you have a financial or academic conflict of interest you should decline the review (as noted above). The rule is full disclosure. If the manuscript originates from your own department (highly unlikely, as most editors will not assign a reviewer from the same institution), this may not constitute a conflict of interest, but it IS something you should disclose.

You will then be asked to rank the manuscript on numeric scales for originality, interest (suitability for the journal), readability, organization/elements, and scientific value. You may be asked if you think statistical review is warranted. You will be asked to rank priority for publication. There will be a box into which you can enter free text "Comments for Authors" and "Comments for Editors." And, finally, you will be asked to recommend "Accept," "reject," or "revise." Sometimes there are two categories of "revise" – "major revision" (also known as "reject and resubmit" or "revise and resubmit") and "minor revision."

We'll deal with the review form last, because it is typically the last thing you work on, but you can view this review form at any step in the process. The review is not finalized until you hit "submit." I do not recommend entering information into the form until you are ready to submit the review; sometimes incomplete reviews fail to save properly.

It is generally most convenient, as well as wise, to enter your comments and critiques into a word-processing program and then paste these blocks of text in the review form.

Information gathering. First, download the manuscript to your computer or smart phone. Print it out if you wish, but in some way ensure that it is accessible in a portable form convenient to you, so that you can read the manuscript at your leisure. Read through it several times – first, do a quick scan, to get a sense of general quality and "publishability."

If the manuscript appears promising (as most will), then do a second, closer read. Note any questions or problems. Either note comments on your manuscript, or put them into a separate computer file.

Second, do a literature search on the topic. Check whether or not recent relevant publications are cited in the work.

Third, search for other publications by the same authors (sometimes the editorial office will already have done this). If an author has published something that seems similar, obtain that paper and check to determine whether you are dealing with duplicate publication.

If you are not familiar with the journal, take the time to learn about it. Go to the journal website and look over typical table of contents. A journal that is read by subspecialists is of necessity going to be different than one read by generalists, and submissions to the two journals will be judged differently. That doesn't mean that substandard work can find a haven in a generalist journal; on the contrary, the standards of some generalist journals (such as the Journal of the American Medical Association) are extremely high; it simply means that the needs and interest and background of the audience may be different.

Many journals will, as part of your review, ask you to rate the manuscript on "interest to our readers." You can only answer this if you have some familiarity with the journal and its mission.

Reading as a reviewer. If you have participated in "Journal Club" you are familiar with the elements of analyzing a paper. Reviewing a paper for potential publication is somewhat similar. What are the stated purposes of the study? What is the study design? Are the methods described in sufficient detail that the motivated reader could replicate the experiment? Are data clearly presented and well-analyzed? Do the data support the conclusions? Are all relevant works cited? Does the title clearly and concisely reflect the content of the paper? What is the quality of the illustrations? Are they all needed, or are other illustrations necessary to clarify technical points? Are graphs and tables clear? Finally, do you suspect this material has been published before (and if so, where)? Is the relevant literature cited and discussed? Make a list of comments as you proceed, and highlight any problematic areas.

When is external statistical review warranted? I generally recommend external statistical review if any but the most basic statistical methodology is being used. Some journals have specific policies on when review is required, and some actually require access to the data on which the manuscript is based. You, as a junior person reading this book, will generally not be operating in those stratospheric levels and in any event, generally this is not done at the reviewer level. In other words, you will not have access to the primary data, just to the manuscript itself.

Completing the review form. When you are ready to actually do the review, log back into the journal site and open the review form. Take care to "save" your review frequently, lest an unreliable internet connection at either end cause difficulties. Be prepared to rank the manuscript on several parameters as previously mentioned. If you have done your preparation well, that will be easy. Near the end you will generally encounter two text boxes. The first one is for "Comments for Authors," and the second is for confidential "Comments for Editors."

By the time you fill out the review form, you should have thought through (and ideally made notes on) the manuscript – its suitability for the journal, its originality, its quality, its strong and weak points – and thus it is just a matter of sitting down and checking off boxes, and entering the "Comments for Authors" and "Comments to the Editors." It is always best to list *all* of your concerns. The experienced editor will be able to discount any that seem overly-picky or irrelevant, and experienced authors will be able to address these easily in their response. It is much harder for the editor to try to figure out why you are recommending "Revise" if your comments/critiques are skimpy or just not helpful.

Strive for clarity in this, as in all writing. Think of an editor, eyes tired, going through a pile of reviewed manuscripts after hours of seeing patients in clinic or standing in the operating room. Think of an author, hopes high, trying to figure out what your critique means.   A comment such as, "The manuscript is sloppily written," may be true but does not help the author as much as giving several examples. Similarly, it is better to list specific examples of conclusions not supported by data than to simply say, "Conclusions are not supported by data."

When I finalize a review, I think of three sets of people to whom I have an obligation: the readers of the journal, the editor of the journal, and the author of the manuscript.

How to write good "Comments for Authors." First of all, you do not need to state the name of the paper or summarize its contents. This formulaic beginning was common in the past, but is no longer used. If it will be helpful in putting your critique in context for the editor, by all means state the nature of the study (e.g "This multicenter prospective clinical trial" or "this single-surgeon retrospective case series") but keep it brief.

This section is now primarily devoted to a numbered list of critiques will help the authors improve the manuscript and will help the editor make a decision. Be as complete as possible; it is far easier for an editor to disregard a critique as overly picky or irrelevant than it is for an editor to figure out why you recommended "accept" or "reject" without any details.

Do not copy-edit the manuscript; it is not your job to point out every typographic error or bad use of English.

I always try to **begin with something positive**, before listing the critiques. There is always something good to say. Be realistic, but compassionate. Remember that a large amount of time, sweat, and toil went into even the worst manuscript, and think about starting with some bland phrase such as "This manuscript represents an attempt to carefully analyze a small series of cases."

Then launch into your unvarnished critique with an introductory phrase such as, "This manuscript would be improved by attention to the following." Strike a balance in your language, so that the author of a doomed manuscript does not get false hope from your first sentences. Make it clear where you stand.

Number your critiques. This allows the author to revise and cite, in their cover letter, how they have addressed each critique by reviewer and by number. Be as specific as possible. Allude to a specific section and line number (provided on most manuscripts). For example, "In the Discussion section, line 2145 draws conclusions not supported by the data." It also helps the authors improve their manuscript before sending it to another journal.

I recommend that you write your comments off-line, using a standard word processing program. That will allow you to edit and spell and grammar-check your comments. You can then copy and paste these into the appropriate block in the form. Your comments will probably similarly be pasted directly into the letter that goes to the author; avoid embarrassment for the editor by making sure that your comments are lucid and well-written.

If the problem is English grammar and usage, do not attempt to correct (or line-edit) the manuscript. Simply note that revision by a native English-speaking writer would be in order.

Some minimal corrections may be needed even if the manuscript originated in the UK for publication in a US journal.

If, through lack of understanding, a sentence or two stand out as totally cryptic or even potentially wrong, it is perfectly fine to quote these as examples. This not only makes your point, but draws the author's attention to a particularly problematic passage. Be sympathetic! Could you write a scientific paper in a language that was not your mother tongue? I could not.

If you feel confident that the manuscript will not merit publication in this particular journal, it is kind to add a sentence suggesting an alternative venue. Something such as, "This manuscript might be more appropriate for a regional journal," or "This manuscript might be more appropriate for an audience of non-specialists," will help give the author some guidance. Generally the reviewer does not name a specific alternate journal, but simply refers to journal type.

How to write good "Comments for Editors." This is the place to be brutally frank, but diplomatic. If you are recommending "reject," it is very helpful to summarize the fatal flaw in the manuscript. Typical fatal flaws include, "Bad science, poorly designed study," "Topic is just not timely," "We do not need another small retrospective study in this area," "Poorly designed study, not salvageable," "More appropriate for a different journal." If you use the latter, explain the audience.

If you think this material has been published before, put a comment to this effect and cite the potential duplicate publication. Duplicate or overlapping publication of the same material is sometimes acceptable; the editor needs all of the facts to make an informed decision.

If you are a senior surgeon, a long-time member of the editorial board and know the editor-in-chief well, you can be less diplomatic and even inject some humor. But if you are reading this book, you are probably a relatively unknown junior surgeon. So, be tactful and humble. It is always possible that this manuscript was submitted by a protégé of the editor and, in any event, senior surgeons rarely appreciate snarky junior colleagues. Just stick to the facts.

On the other hand, if you recommend "accept," it is also important to explain to the editor why you do not think the manuscript could be improved upon. This is a rare recommendation, since most manuscripts go through at least one revision before publication, and a comment justifying your lack of critiques is important.

How to review a revised manuscript. If you have recommended revision, you may be asked to review the revision. Sometimes the original reviewers are not available and you may be asked to review a revised manuscript when you did not perform the original review. In any event, stick to the critique and comments from the editor-in-chief. It is unfair to the author to introduce new problems at this stage. Very rarely, as a reviewer new to the manuscript, you may spot a fatal flaw that previous reviewers missed. In this situation, carefully document your concerns in the "Comments to the Editor" section of the review form.

Generally the decision at this point is "accept" or "reject." Under exceptional circumstances, an additional revision may be required from the authors. Your job, therefore, is to determine whether each critique was addressed. The journal will usually supply you with the decision letter that provides the complete critique. It will also give you a letter from the authors addressing each point in the critique. Finally, you will have the revised (and usually also the original) manuscript and search engine access.

Remember that the point of the whole exercise is to improve the manuscript. Each item in the critique must be addressed in the manuscript, not just in the response letter. Contradictory critiques from different reviewers can occur, but usually mean that something is just not clear in the manuscript. The wise author will recognize and revise that section for clarity.

Special circumstances. Some surgical meetings have arrangements with specific journals and a certain number of pages are reserved by the journal for papers from the meeting. The first review of submitted papers is typically performed by senior members of the association sponsoring the meeting. A second review is then performed by the journal editor in the usual fashion. If you are a member of the publications committee, or the program committee, or the executive committee, or in some other leadership capacity, you may be asked to perform this first review. Often this is done during the meeting. The primary differences between this kind of review and the normal review is that the timeline is particularly tight, you may be asked to review a cluster of manuscripts (as many as six or more) from the meeting at the same time, and the page count may be tight.

Last words. The manuscript is confidential. When you are done with your review, destroy all copies. Do not share the manuscript with anyone. The single exception to the rule might be a colleague more experienced in the area than yourself – if so, check with the editorial office first. Finally, do not copy any of the ideas or words – this is plagiarism.

References

Durning SJ, Carline JD, eds. Review Criteria for Research Manuscripts, 2nd ed. Washington, DC: Association of American Medical Colleges; 2015. Available for download as a free .pdf file through the AAMC website: www.aamc.org (under "Publications") or from this URL: https://members.aamc.org/eweb/DynamicPage.aspx?Action=Add &ObjectKeyFrom=1A83491A-9853-4C87-86A4-F7D95601C2E2&WebCode=PubDetailAdd&DoNotSave=yes&Pa rentObject=CentralizedOrderEntry&ParentDataObject=Invoice% 20Detail&ivd_formkey=69202792-63d7-4ba2-bf4e-a0da41270555&ivd_prc_prd_key=3CCCBB8D-BB9A-4794-A2C2-E6E1A6F0D421.

Hames I (on behalf of COPE Council), March 2013, v.1. COPE Ethical Guidelines for Peer Reviewers. Available at: www.publicationethics.org (http://www.publicationethics.org/).

Chapter 13. The View from the Editorial Office

This chapter discusses the editorial office from two viewpoints: first of all, how does one get involved with editorial boards of journals; and, second, what are the concerns of the editor-in-chief. As you begin your career, a position on an editorial board or the office of editor-in- chief may seem unattainable. Remember, just as you had to learn how to operate and take care of patients, and you are now learning how to write, editors learn and earn their craft and positions. I hope this brief overview will whet your enthusiasm and maybe give some further insights into the process.

How to Get Started

Journals may, from time to time, ask you to review manuscripts. The previous chapter discussed in detail how to go about this and the pros and cons of accepting an assignment.

While a solid reputation as a reliable reviewer is not sufficient to get you onto an editorial board, a bad reputation (that is, this person refuses manuscripts, doesn't follow through and submit reviews, is always late, reviews are not helpful – and so on) can easily torpedo you. Journals keep statistics on reviewers, and the input of the managing editor or editorial assistant (the person who actually handles the flow of manuscripts) can be crucial.

If a journal is housed in your institution, introduce yourself to the editorial assistant and the editor-in-chief and volunteer for any needed tasks. Often there is something that needs to be done that the editor-in-chief has not yet assigned. Suggest a new way of reaching the readership. As I write this, "Twitter Journal Clubs" are being established at a variety of journals. This highly successful concept sprung from a suggestion by a relatively young physician who was more familiar with the use of social media than the rest of the editorial board.

If you do not have an editorial office housed in your department, scan the editorial "masthead" of several journals in your field of specialization and look for mentors, people you trained under, and so on. Ideally you want to find an editor-in-chief with whom you have some connection. Contact this person and volunteer, just as suggested above. There is a lot of work to be done on a journal editorial board, and willing and capable workers are rarely turned away.

This is an area where your relative youth is actually an advantage. Most editorial board members (and essentially all editors-in-chief) have attained their position through years of solid scholarly achievement. The more prestigious the journal, the more senior the members of the editorial board tend to be. Yet one of the key issues for any journal is how to fulfill the needs of its current readers and to reach out to new ones. In particular, journals want to build readership among young physicians. You have a far greater first-hand knowledge of how younger readers access information than the senior editorial staff has, and this expertise can be of immeasurable help to the editorial board.

Do not take rejection personally. Be patient. But if you *are* given an assignment as a junior person, put a full effort into earning your place.

Be wary of invitations that seem "too good to be true." If you, as a relatively junior person, receive an e-mail inviting you to join the editorial board of a journal (often electronic) you have never heard of, be wary. Check with some senior colleagues and consult a medical reference librarian to determine if the position will be worth the time involved. Your name on the editorial masthead (with your institutional affiliation) may be lending credibility to a so-called "predatory open access" journal (see http://scholarlyoa.com/). Open Access journals are discussed further in Chapter 2.

What Does the Editorial Board Do?

The members of the editorial board serve as advisors to the editor-in-chief. Often an editorial board is carefully composed to provide complete coverage of subjects (areas of expertise), geography (e.g. international editors from countries that are actively involved with the journal or are areas of potential interest to the journal), and affiliated associations.

The editorial board typically meets once a year in conjunction with a major national or international meeting. Thus, many surgery journals hold editorial board meetings during the Fall Clinical Congress of the American College of Surgeons.

At that meeting, the editor-in-chief and a representative from the publisher present statistics about journal performance (see sections which follow) and solicit input from the board. These meetings are useful brainstorming sessions. Most of the work of the board is done outside the annual meeting, however.

Editorial Board members are expected to review manuscripts. These will generally be manuscripts in their particular area of interest, but sometimes "difficult to place" manuscripts are assigned to editorial board members. As an editorial board member you can expect to review 20-30 manuscripts per year.

You may also be asked to help solicit more manuscripts, by identifying topics for invited reviews or by helping to target authors who have presented good information at meetings but will not have published a manuscript. To this end, some Editorial Boards give business cards to their board members, with the intent that the member will hand these out to likely authors at national and international meetings.

Specialized Roles within the Editorial Board

Some specialized positions that might appeal to a younger physician include: new technology editor, book review editor, video editor, or editor for social media. To look at just one of these positions, the Book Review editor receives newly published books on behalf of the journal. These books are then sent out for review, and the editor collates, edits, and submits these for publication.

Serving as Editor-in-Chief of a Journal

This is typically an opportunity that comes after years of service and experience. Some journals conduct a national search; others rely on a publications committee of the parent organization. Most editors are self-taught, or come to the chief position after years as an associate or assistant to the editor-in-chief. The formal editorial office of the journal may be located at the parent institution of the editor-in-chief, with some variable degree of financial support for operating expenses. While a large prestigious journal may pay the editor-in-chief a stipend, many smaller journals do not.

The journal will require a great deal of work. The editor-in-chief, typically in conjunction with an editorial assistant or managing editor, receives all submitted manuscripts. There is generally some kind of initial triage to assure that the manuscript is worth sending out for review.

If the manuscript appears to meet the criteria established by the journal (topic, length, format, readability) it is sent out for peer review. Three reviewers are selected from the editorial board or from databases kept by the journal. Sometimes specialists who have written papers in the area are identified through a PubMed search. Invitations are sent out and reviews accumulated. A final decision is then rendered.

When all goes well, the three peer reviewers agree to review the manuscript and submit their reviews on time. Typically, however, one or two of the reviewers refuse the initial assignment. Or, even worse, they accept the assignment but never complete the review. Meanwhile the clock is ticking, as most journals pride themselves on a fast decision and rapid publication of accepted manuscripts (called "turnaround). The editorial assistant generally keeps track of the progress of individual manuscripts as well as the aggregate performance of the journal, and advises the editor-in-chief of status several times a week.

The editor-in-chief can expect to need to identify alternate reviewers and most experienced editors will invite three from a possible field of four or five. A minimum of two and preferably three peer reviews are used to formulate the final decision.

That decision will range from "Accept as is" through "Reject." If significant concerns are received from the reviewers the editor-in-chief may decide to reject. If the critiques indicate that the manuscript has promise, the author may be asked to revise and resubmit. Typically, as noted in chapter 10, reviewers disagree. Sometimes, in this situation, another reviewer is invited – typically a member of the editorial board who is known for good reviews on a fast turnaround.

The editor-in-chief assembles manuscripts for each issue, sometimes grouping them around a specific topic. A balance must be maintained between rapid turnaround (time to publication) and a kind of "buffer capacity" that insures each issue can be filled and sent out on time.

In addition to the daily routine of keeping the manuscripts flowing and assembling each issue, the editor-in-chief needs to strategically support and build the journal. This involves a lot more than just soliciting the best manuscripts obtainable. Alliances may be sought with various small specialty associations to create arrangements where a certain number of pages in one issue may be devoted to papers from the annual meeting. Such an arrangement may include a subscription to the journal for the association members. The publisher helps with the logistics and cost-accounting of various arrangements.

The editor-in-chief and publisher closely track the Impact Factor and work to increase it by publishing the best and most citable papers.

Other Concerns of the Editor-in-Chief

Editors-in-chief are very concerned with issues of fraudulent and duplicate publication. In essence, the peer review system relies on a certain element of trust. A PubMed search on the keyword "retraction" will pull scores of papers that have been retracted by the journal in which they were published.

Common reasons for retraction include fraud, duplicate publication, and frank plagiarism from another author. The retraction note becomes linked with the original article electronically. In the stacks of medical libraries where print journals are still housed, a librarian stamps the retracted article with a special stamp so that no one is deceived.

Undisclosed conflict of interest, both financial and non-financial is another major concern. Unfortunately, sometimes this emerges after a paper is published. An erratum, addendum, or even (in severe cases) a retraction may be appropriate.

This is obviously a very black mark on the author, and journals do not do this lightly. Authors sometimes threaten legal action, another concern for the editor-in-chief!
With all of these concerns, you might wonder why anyone takes the job. It's simple. Editors-in-chief love writing, love their work, and love getting well-written and publishable manuscripts.

Chapter 14. Useful Tools

This chapter gathers into one place various tools mentioned earlier in the text. While these may seem like gimmicks, they are all useful tactics that have worked for other beginning writers.

Manuscript Log

A manuscript log is simply a way to track progress on each particular project. It is used to monitor deadlines, and is particularly helpful during the abstract and manuscript submission process. The log can be an actual physical notebook, or an electronic database. I have found that a spiral-bound notebook works well.

When you start a new project, start a new page (an entry) in your log. That entry includes the following basic information:

- Title (proposed)
- Authors and their roles
- Relevant deadlines – abstract submission, manuscript due

As you work on the manuscript, make additional entries to track the progress.

Suppose, for example, that you have sent your manuscript out to coauthors for review and comment. Give them a deadline and make this a log entry. When the manuscript is ready to submit, add the following information:

- Name of journal and date submitted
- Date of rejection or request for revision
- Date revision submitted
- Final disposition
- Name of second choice journal

When a manuscript is accepted for publication, celebrate by marking the date of acceptance. In my physical notebook, I fold the page in half so that only the active projects stand out. There is a lot of satisfaction in folding the page over.

Whiteboard

A whiteboard is a simple but effective time-management aid. It is basically a very high-level "to do" list spanning the next six to twelve months. Enumerate all of your major projects – research grants, papers to write, chapters that you have promised, forthcoming presentations, proposals that are due and so on. List the target dates for completion of each one.

Make the whiteboard work for you. Some people list everything in a simple chronologic order. Others cluster tasks by type, listing presentations, papers, and research grant proposals in different columns. However you choose to list things, create a system that helps you see the next six months or year at a glance. Cross things off as you accomplish them. Keep your whiteboard in easy sight as a reminder of the larger picture – what you seek to accomplish this academic year.

Task List

Break down each project into small tasks. Be as specific as possible, and enter these on your personal schedule. Thus, instead of blocking off one hour on Saturday to "work on manuscript," identify the next logical task and a step that you can do in the available time. Such steps might include "Revise discussion," or "Reword paragraph 2 of discussion to address critique _____." Make your task list as specific as you might have made your scut list during residency.

When you assign tasks to your coauthors, be as specific as possible and give them a deadline. If possible, phrase your request so that failure to respond is assumed to be agreement. For example, if you want your coauthors to review and comment on the final version of the manuscript, you might phrase your detailed request and end with a sentence such as, "If I do not hear from you by _____, I will assume that you have no changes to recommend."

Abstract Submission Deadline Calendar

Presenting material at regional, national, and international meetings is a great way to gain visibility and may lead to publication. Make this easy by tracking key dates including:

- Abstract submissions date
- Notification date
- Date of meeting (and whether or not a manuscript is expected

Although meeting and abstract submission dates tend to vary a bit from year to year, these will generally occur at around the same time of year. For example, the San Antonio Breast Cancer Symposium meets in early December and has its abstract submission deadline in June. This is a pretty typical pattern in that abstracts are due six months before the meeting.

You can use an electronic calendar, or a simple printed calendar (the kind that you hang on the wall, with a page for each month). It is still a lot easier just to write notes on a wall calendar. Use the same calendar for several years. Concentrate on month and date – the day of the week is irrelevant. You will start to see patterns, and that helps you anticipate and plan.

Start your abstract submission calendar by making a note on this calendar every time a "call for abstracts" comes out. Note these dates:

- Call for abstracts received for ___ meeting
- Abstract submission deadline for ___ meeting
- Notification date for ___ meeting
- Date of the meeting.

Also note whether or not a manuscript will be expected at that time. You will soon find that meetings tend to cluster in the spring and the fall (with some notable exceptions such as the meeting cited above).

Make note of the "notification date" as well. This date will be about two months after the submission deadline.

As you compile your calendar over the next year or two, you will start to see possibilities. For example, you may note that an enticing abstract deadline is coming up and you can complete your data analysis in time to submit an abstract. You also see that the notification date will allow you to submit to another really good meeting that will be sending out a call for abstracts shortly thereafter, in case your first choice rejects the abstract.

Of course, just as with manuscript submission, you generally cannot submit to multiple meetings at once, or present data at more than one meeting.

Handling your Manuscript

Always back up your files. Save changes as you make them. Assign each manuscript a title that will make it easy for you to

118

retrieve it. Avoid generic titles like "chapter" or "paper" or "abstract." Believe it or not, you will write more than one of these.

Some writers save every revision as a separate file. Most prefer to simply overwrite the old files, unless a major revision (for example, in response to a colleague's review or a journal's critiques) is performed. If you are fortunate enough to have a colleague willing to make specific changes and suggestions, save that marked up (either hardcopy or electronic) version in a special file. Use this specific example (and others, as you accumulate them) to improve your writing skills.

Electronic formats change. During my writing career, I've seen the development of word processing software, seen such software come and go, and gone through innumerable personal computers and storage formats. There is no substitute for keeping a clean, double-spaced printout of your final manuscript in a file.

Writing mentors, partners, and groups

You are not the only struggling writer out there. Reach out and find others who can help you. Many departments house experienced faculty who love to write and who are willing to read and/or edit manuscripts for beginners. Do not simply incorporate all of their suggested changes. Study how their revisions change the language and flow of your writing. Keep copies of their comments, so that you can study what they did. You will start to notice patterns. Try to anticipate and obey their most common suggestions, thus internalizing their advice, and you will improve your writing style.

Look for mentors in unexpected places. A laboratory technician, for example, may have a strong writing background and be just the person you need to tighten up your prose.

Check with faculty development at your institution and see if there is a writing group that you can join. If none exists, consider forming one. Often a medical school or department will, if asked, sponsor such a group – providing meeting space, minimal administrative support (to schedule meetings and e-mail the participants), and sometimes even refreshments.

Writing groups are a common strategy for creative writers. With some minimal changes, the concept has been adapted to the needs of medical writers. Such groups meet on a weekly or monthly basis and generally review/critique one manuscript at each meeting. Sometimes this is done as a virtual meeting. An excellent article in The Chronicle of Higher Education tells how one successful academic writing group operates (http://chronicle.com/article/The-Rules-of-Writing-Group/126880/). Key concepts include:

- Find a small group of congenial and trustworthy writers
- Schedule a block of time to meet
- Attend and participate in meetings
- Circulate your own writing when it is your turn
- Read and thoughtfully (and constructively) comment on others' submissions

A writing group is a safe space in which writers explore and grow together. It can be as few as three writers, or as large as 8-10. Small groups are often extremely successful and larger groups less so (perhaps because each member of a large group thinks the other members will do what needs to be done).

Chapter 15. Additional Recommended Resources

Here are some resources that may be helpful. Many are cited in the previous chapters. They are collected here in one place for your convenience. I've included a brief reason for inclusion to help guide you.

I have included URLs for your convenience. These URLs were functional as of October 2015. If you find that a link is broken, try entering the name of the particular resource or sponsoring organization into a search engine.

Books – There are a lot of books on medical writing and medical research. These go into specific topics in greater depth. Here are three that I have found particularly useful to beginners.

- **Browner WS. "Publishing and Presenting Clinical Research." 3rd edition, 2012, Lippincott Williams & Wilkins, Philadelphia PA.** This is a comprehensive and highly readable yet compact paperback. It deals exclusively with clinical research, but it goes far beyond writing and devotes chapters to "Authorship," "Posters," and "Oral Presentations." It gives wonderful tips for how to prepare a poster and what to do when you find yourself standing alone in front of your poster for the first time. It gives examples of how to respond to discussants during an oral presentation. Perhaps most helpful of all, it includes sample scripts for *very* thorny situations – for example, how to tell your boss he/she does not deserve to have his/her name added to your paper.
- **Byrne DW. "Publishing your Medical Research Paper. What They Don't Teach You in Medical School." 1998, Lippincott Williams & Wilkins, Philadelphia PA.** This comprehensive paperback is

divided into three sections. The first two, "Planning" and "Observing," deal with research design and data analysis. The third, "Writing," is self-explanatory. A chapter entitled "Preparing to Write a Publishable Paper" deals with identifying significant issues to research. It may be of particular value to beginners.

- **Taylor RB. "The Clinician's Guide to Medical Writing." 2005, Springer Verlag, New York.** This is nice compact text that delves into selected topics in greater detail. The author is a distinguished leader in academic family medicine. About half of this paperback is devoted to general writing advice and strategies, and the other half includes specific chapters on Review Articles, Case Reports, Book Chapters, and results of Clinical Studies.

- **Tufte ER. The Visual Display of Quantitative Information. 2001. Connecticut. Graphics Press.** This is a classic and elegant text that explains how graphs and other images can represent and clarify, or misrepresent and confuse, information. It is a delight to read. The author followed with several additional texts, but this is the classic one.

- **Strunk W, White EB. The Elements of Style. 4th edition, 1999, Longmen.** You may have read this one in college. Read it again. Clarity of writing is the essence of good style.

- **Broad W, Wade N. Betrayers of the Truth: Fraud and Deceit in the Halls of Science.** 1983. New York NY. Simon & Shuster. Sobering account of actual fraud, and, more importantly, ways in which conscious and unconscious bias can alter the results of scientific studies.

Academic Career Development Resources

- **Chen H, Kao LS. "Success in Academic Surgery"2012, Springer Verlag, New York NY.** This is a slim multiauthored paperback largely authored by members of the Association for Academic Surgery. While aimed at surgeons, there is a lot of generally good advice here.

- **Pories SE et al (editors) "Navigating Your Surgical Career: The AWS Guide to Success" 2015, The Association of Women Surgeons.** This is available through their website (https://www.womensurgeons.org/) and from online booksellers. You don't have to be a woman to benefit from the advice in this book. Includes both academic career development and general leadership advice.

Sources of Guidelines

- **The International Committee of Medical Journal Editors** – Uniform, agreed-upon, guidelines for authorship, overlapping publications, peer review, and a variety of other important topics (http://www.icmje.org/).
- **CARE** – Case Report guidelines (http://www.care-statement.org/)
- **Cochrane Collaborative Guidelines** - How to perform a Cochrane review (http://www.cochranelibrary.com/help/how-to-prepare-a-cochrane-review.html).
- **Cochrane Collaborative Handbook** – More detailed information on systematic reviews and meta-analyses (http://handbook.cochrane.org/).
- **CONSORT (Consolidated Standards of Reporting Trials)** – Guidelines and a checklist for reporting clinical trials (http://www.consort-statement.org/).
- **COPE (The Committee on Publication Ethics)** – Guidelines on a variety of publication ethics topics, including peer review (http://publicationethics.org/resources/guidelines).

- **AAMC Review Criteria** – Peer review guidelines from the American Association of Medical Colleges (http://publicationethics.org/files/Ethical_guidelines_for _peer_reviewers_0.pdf).

Other Useful Sites

- **Impact Factor**– Information about how journals are ranked (http://wokinfo.com/essays/impact-factor/).
- **Public Library of Science (PLOS)** - Information about "open access" journals (https://www.plos.org/open-access/).
- **Medical Subject Headings (MeSH)** – standard key words and phrases that facilitate retrieval of your article through PubMed searches (https://www.nlm.nih.gov/mesh/).
- **NBME® (National Board of Medical Examiners) Item-Writing Handbook** – How to write good multiple choice questions (http://www.nbme.org/publications/item-writing-manual.html).
- **JANE or Journal/Author Name Estimator** – A search engine that allows you to enter a title, or even a complete abstract, and find journals that publish similar material (http://www.biosemantics.org/jane/).
- **The Association of Medical Illustrators** – The professional organization for illustrators. Their website includes an excellent set of "Client Guidelines" (http://ami.org/professional-resources/client-guide).
- **Scholarly Open Access** – A site that monitors "predatory open access publishers." This site maintains (somewhat controversial) lists of predatory publishers and journals (http://scholarlyoa.com/).

CPSIA information can be obtained
at www.ICGtesting.com
Printed in the USA
LVHW05090525042O
654389LV00005B/416